P9-EJO-363

THE SOUTH BEACH DIET

A Doctor's Plan for Fast and Lasting Weight Loss

Dr A. Agatston

headline

This publication constitutes an exclusive abridgement of
The South Beach Diet by Dr Arthur Agatston for *Cosmopolitan*
magazine. The full edition, including all recipes, is published by
Headline Book Publishing, priced £10.99.

First published in Great Britain in 2003
by HEADLINE BOOK PUBLISHING

Published by arrangement with Rodale, Inc., Emmaus, PA, USA

10 9 8 7 6 5 4 3 2 1

ISBN 0 7553 1301 1

Typeset in Gill Sans by
Letterpart Limited, Reigate, Surrey

Printed and bound in Great Britain by
Mackays of Chatham plc, Chatham, Kent

Every effort has been made to fulfil requirements
with regard to reproducing copyright material.
The author and publisher will be glad to rectify
any omissions at the earliest opportunity.

Papers and cover board used by Headline are natural, recyclable products
made from wood grown in sustainable forests. The manufacturing processes
conform to the environmental regulations of the country of origin.

HEADLINE BOOK PUBLISHING
A division of Hodder Headline
338 Euston Road
LONDON NW1 3BH

www.headline.co.uk
www.hodderheadline.com

contents

introduction

Repeat after me: 'I love my body the way it is'; 'I love my tummy, my thighs, my bottom, however they look'. No matter how many times you look in the mirror and say this, you probably still won't be happy with your body. Some women are lucky – they are able to love their shape regardless, and I applaud them. How I wish we could all be like that. But, realistically, millions of women are not happy with their shape. We want to lose weight. We want to be slimmer, feel fitter and be healthier. At *Cosmopolitan* it is our job to help you be the best you can be, to give you the advice and information you need to feel happy and secure in your day-to-day life, which is why I didn't make the decision to give you a diet book lightly. But we realised that so many of you desperately wanted us to help you lose weight. That's why, after months of looking at many different diets, we have finally found the one which was medically, emotionally and practically suitable for young women today. This authoritative book has been written by a heart doctor. It is not a dangerous, faddy food book that will be impossible to follow. It is simple to understand and non-constricting – it is more of an eating plan than a calorie-controlled diet. It doesn't involve complicated portion measuring or difficult recipes. This diet is not about denial or a lifetime of longing for a sweet treat. It's about rethinking the way you eat – and then enjoying your food more. It's completely safe and, if you follow it properly, you will lose weight forever. If you are happy with the weight you are, that's brilliant. If not, this book will help you get the new body you want. There is no perfect weight or perfect shape. And we don't promise that by being slimmer, any emotional dilemmas you face will be cured. But if losing weight makes you happier and healthier, this excellent book is for you. Good luck!

Lorraine Candy
Editor *Cosmopolitan*

losing weight
gaining life

part I

Understanding the
South Beach Diet

losing weight, gaining life

The South Beach Diet is not low carb. Nor is it low fat.

The South Beach Diet teaches you to rely on the right carbs and the right fats – the *good* ones – and enables you to live quite happily without the bad carbs and bad fats. As a result, you're going to get healthy and lose weight – somewhere between 8 and 13 pounds in the next two weeks alone.

Here's how you'll do it.

You'll eat normal-size helpings of meat, chicken, turkey, fish, and shellfish.

You'll have plenty of vegetables. Eggs. Cheese. Nuts.

You'll have salads with real olive oil in the dressing.

You'll have three balanced meals a day, and it will be your job to eat so that your hunger is satisfied. Nothing undermines a weight-loss plan more than the distressing sensation that you need more food. No sane eating programme expects you to go through life feeling discomfort. You'll be urged to have snacks in the mid-morning and mid-afternoon, whether you need to or not. You'll have dessert after dinner.

You'll drink water, of course, plus coffee or tea if you wish.

For the next 14 days you *won't* be having any bread, rice, potatoes, pasta, or baked goods. No fruit, even. Before you panic: You'll begin adding those things back into your diet again in two weeks. But for right now, they're off-limits.

No sweets, cake, biscuits, or ice-cream for two weeks, either. No beer or alcohol of any kind. After this phase you'll be free to drink wine. It's beneficial for a variety of reasons. Not a drop to drink during the first two weeks, however.

Now, if you're the kind of person who lives for pasta or bread or potatoes, or if you believe that you can't get through a day without feeding your sweet tooth (three or four times), let me tell you something: You're going to be shocked at how painlessly two weeks without these foods will pass. The first day or two may be challenging, but once you weather that you'll be fine. It's not that you'll have to fight your urges – during the first week the cravings will virtually disappear. I say this with such confidence only because it's what so many overweight people who have already succeeded on this programme tell me. The South Beach Diet may be new to you, but it has existed for several years, long enough to have helped hundreds of people lose weight easily and keep it off.

So that's Phase 1, the strictest period.

After two weeks of that, you will be somewhere between 9 and 13 pounds lighter than you are today. Most of that weight will come off your mid-section, so right away you'll notice the difference in your clothes. It will be easier to zip your jeans than it's been for some time. That blazer will close without a bulge.

But this will just be the noticeable difference. You won't be able to see that during those two weeks you'll also have changed yourself internally. You will have corrected the way your body reacts to the very foods that made you overweight. There's a switch inside you that had been turned on. Now, simply by modifying your diet, you'll have turned it off. The physical cravings that ruled your eating habits will be gone, and they'll stay away for as long as you stick with the programme. The weight loss doesn't happen because you're trying to eat less. But you'll be eating fewer of the foods that created those bad old urges, fewer of the foods that caused your body to store excessive fat.

As a result of *that* change, you will continue losing weight after the 14-day period ends, even though by then you will have begun adding some of those banished foods back into your life. You'll still be on a diet, but if it's bread you love, you'll have bread. If it's pasta, you'll reintroduce that. Rice or cereal, too. Potatoes. Fruit will definitely be back.

Chocolate? If it makes you feel good, sure. You will have to pick and choose which of these indulgences you permit yourself. You won't be able to have them all, all the time. You'll learn to enjoy them a little differently than before – maybe a little less enthusiastically. But you will enjoy them again soon.

That's Phase 2.

You'll remain in that phase and continue losing weight until you reach your goal. How long it takes depends on how much you need to lose. In Phase 2 people lose, on average, a pound or two a week. Once you hit your target, you'll switch to an even more liberal version of the programme, which will help you to maintain your ideal weight.

That's Phase 3.

That stage is the one that lasts the rest of your life. When you get to that point, you'll notice that this plan feels less like a diet and more like a way of life – you'll be eating normal foods, after all, in normal-size portions. You can then feel free to forget all about the South Beach Diet, as long as you remember to live by its few basic rules.

As you're losing weight and altering how your body responds to food, a third change will be taking place. This one will significantly alter your blood chemistry, to the long-term benefit of your cardiovascular system. You will improve invisible factors that only cardiologists and heart patients worry about. Thanks to this final change, you will substantially increase your odds of living long and well – meaning, you will maintain your health and vitality as you age.

You may start on the South Beach Diet hoping just to lose weight. If you adopt it and stay with it, you will surely accomplish that much. But you'll also do a lot more for yourself, all of it very good. I'm not exaggerating when I say that this diet can, as a fringe benefit, save your life.

good carbs, bad carbs

I'm not a diet doctor.

In fact, my career in medicine has been largely devoted to the science of non-invasive cardiac imaging – the development of technology that produces sophisticated pictures of the heart and the coronary blood vessels. This allows us to identify problems and treat them early, before they cause heart attack or stroke. In CT (computerized tomography) scanning all over the world, I'm proud to say, the measure of coronary calcium is called the Agatston Score, and the protocol for calcium screening is often referred to as the Agatston Method. I maintain an active, full-time cardiology practice, both clinical and research.

So how is it I am also responsible for a weight-loss programme that has become a phenomenon in South Florida – a regime that's helped countless women and men, many of them in their twenties and thirties, young enough to be the grandchildren of my usual cardiology patients – get down to string bikini and Speedo swimming trunks shape?

I have to admit, I wasn't prepared to find myself on the receiving end of so much buzz. I'm now regularly stopped by people who have seen my TV news appearances or read about the diet's success in newspapers and magazines. Given South Beach's worldwide image as a mecca of physical beauty and body consciousness and its role as a chic outpost of the fashion industry, it's an unexpected position to find myself in.

This all started, however, as a serious medical undertaking. Back in the mid-nineties I was but one of many cardiologists who had grown disillusioned with the low-fat, high-carbohydrate diet recommended by the American

Heart Association in order to help us all eat properly and maintain healthy weight. None of the low-fat regimes of that era seemed to work reliably, especially over the long haul. My concern was not with my patients' appearance, of course: I wanted to find a diet that would help prevent or reverse the myriad heart and vascular problems that stem from obesity.

I never found such a diet. Instead, I developed it myself.

Today, I feel nearly as comfortable in the world of nutrition as I do among cardiologists. I speak regularly before physicians, researchers, and other health-care professionals who devote their lives to helping patients eat sensibly and lose weight. Although my interest in diet started from the therapeutic perspective, I see now that the cosmetic benefits of losing weight are extremely important because they so effectively motivate the young *and* the old – even more than the promise of a healthy heart, it often seems. The psychological lift that comes from an improved appearance benefits the entire person, and in turn keeps many a patient from backsliding – which, in the end, benefits cardiovascular health, my only goal when this journey began.

What started as a part-time foray into the world of nutrition has led me to devise a simple, medically sound diet that works, without stress, for a large percentage of those who try it, a programme that has been scientifically studied (as few diets ever are) and proven effective both for losing weight and for getting and keeping a healthy cardiovascular system.

Back when this all began, of course, I had no idea what would ensue. All I knew was that many of my patients – more of them every year – were overweight and that their condition was a big part of their cardiac burden. I could treat them with all the newest medications and procedures, but until they got their diet under control we were often fighting a losing battle. Their eating habits contributed to blood chemistry that was dangerously high in cholesterol and triglycerides, the leading factors in blocked arteries and inflammation of the blood vessels. And there was another, not terribly well-understood diet-related problem that they shared, a silent, so-called *metabolic* syndrome (prediabetes) found in close to half of all Americans who suffer heart attacks.

Searching for the right weight-loss plan

My journey to disease prevention through diet actually began when my education as a cardiologist did, 30 years ago. During my training in the late

1970s, I looked forward to treating patients with heart disease – despite the fact that we didn't have many preventative weapons in our arsenal. I asked the most respected cardiologist I knew this question: 'What is the best way to prevent heart disease?' His answer: 'Pick the right parents.' If you inherited the gene for cardiac longevity, you were likely to live to a ripe old age. If heart disease struck early in your family, there was not much you could do to change your destiny.

Then, in 1984, I attended a course at the Heart House in Bethesda, Maryland, the national headquarters of the American College of Cardiology. There, I heard a lecture by a brilliant researcher and charismatic teacher, Bill Castelli, who headed the world-famous Framingham Heart Study. Dr Castelli told us about the results of the recently completed National Institutes of Health (NIH)-sponsored Lipid Research Clinics Primary Prevention Trial (LRCPPT). This was the very first study to prove that lowering cholesterol via diet could reduce heart attacks. At the time, the only known treatment for high cholesterol was an unpleasant, grainy powder known as a resin, which was taken several times a day before meals. Therefore, we were all very excited when Dr Castelli told the conference that if we put patients on the very first American Heart Association diet, we could lower their cholesterol and end the scourge of heart disease in America.

We physicians all returned home filled with fervour, ready to guide our patients to restored cardiac health and dietary wisdom. I came back to Miami confident in my newfound knowledge of how to save my patients' lives. My wife and I even joked that with heart disease out of the picture, I might be better off switching to a growth specialty, like plastic surgery. It wasn't long before I learned that unemployment as a cardiologist was going to be unlikely.

I began counselling my patients on the low-fat, high-carbohydrate diet advocated by the American Heart Association, but the results fell far below my expectations. Often, there was an initial modest improvement in total cholesterol with mild weight loss. This invariably was followed by a return of cholesterol to its previous level or higher, along with a return of the lost weight. This scenario was not only my experience but also that of my colleagues. It was reflected in the many diet-cholesterol trials documented in the literature that showed our inability to sustain cholesterol and/or weight reductions using low-fat, high-carbohydrate diets. There were no convincing studies showing that the American Heart Association diet saved lives.

Over the years I had suggested most of the highly respected diets out there – going back to Pritikin (see chapter three) and then through the various, more recent, heart-healthy low-fat regimes, including the Ornish plan and several American Heart Association diets – and seen each of them, for different reasons, fail miserably. Either the diets were too difficult to stick with, or the promise of improved blood chemistry and cardiac health remained just that – a promise. Discouraged, I had all but given up on advising my patients about nutrition, because I was unable to suggest anything that actually helped. Like most cardiologists in that period, I turned instead to the statin drugs that were just coming on the market, medications that had proven extremely effective in lowering total cholesterol, if not weight.

But I also decided, as a last-ditch effort, that I would devote some serious study of my own to diet and obesity. Like most physicians, I was not particularly knowledgeable in the science of nutrition. So my first task was to research all the weight-loss programmes out there, the serious scientific ones as well as the trendy attempts that topped the best-seller lists. As I acquired that education, I was also reading in the cardiology literature about the prevalence of something called the insulin resistance syndrome and its effect on obesity and heart health.

The science of success

One side effect of excess weight, we now know, is an impairment of the hormone insulin's ability to do its job of processing fuel, or fats and sugars, properly. This condition is commonly called insulin resistance. As a result, the body stores more fat than it should, especially in the mid-section. We've been genetically conditioned to store fat since the dawn of *homo sapiens*, as a survival strategy to see us through times of famine.

The problem now, of course, is that we never experience the famine end of that equation, only the feast. As a result, we store fat but never require our bodies to burn it off. Much of our excess weight comes from the carbohydrates we eat, especially the highly processed ones found in baked goods, breads, snacks, and other convenient favourites. Modern industrial processing removes the fibre from these foods, and once that's gone their very nature – and how we metabolize them – changes significantly, and for the worse.

Decrease the consumption of those 'bad' carbs, studies showed, and the insulin resistance starts clearing up on its own. Weight begins a fairly rapid decrease, and you begin metabolizing carbs properly. Even the craving for carbs disappears once you cut down on their consumption. Finally, cutting out processed carbs improves blood chemistry, ultimately resulting in lowered triglycerides and cholesterol.

So my eating plan's first principle was to permit good carbohydrates (fruits, vegetables, and whole grains) and curtail the intake of bad carbohydrates (the highly processed ones, for the most part, where all the fibre had been stripped away during manufacturing). We would thereby eliminate a prime cause of obesity. This was in marked contrast to the Atkins Diet, for instance, which bans virtually *all* carbohydrates and leaves the dieter to exist mostly on proteins. That regime also permits limitless saturated fats, the kind found in red meat and butter. These are, as most people know, the bad fats – the ones that can lead to cardiovascular disease, heart attack, and stroke. That hasn't stopped millions of dieters from adopting the plan. But from the moment I learned of it, the diet set off alarm bells in this cardiologist's head. Even if you do lose weight and keep it off, your blood chemistry is bound to suffer from eating so much saturated fat.

My plan cut certain carbohydrates, but not all. In fact, it encouraged eating the good ones. For instance, I banished white flour and white sugar. But our diet permits whole grain breads and cereals and wholemeal pasta. We also prescribe lots of vegetables and fruit. I had a practical reason, beyond their obvious nutritional value and the beneficial fibre they provide, for that decision. Not everyone *wants* to give up vegetables, fruit, bread, and pasta for ever, even in exchange for a regime that allows a pound of bacon for breakfast, followed by a pound of hamburger (with no bun, of course) for lunch, topped by a thick steak for dinner. And if people want bread, pasta, or rice, a humane eating plan should be able to accommodate that desire.

To make up for the overall cut in carbohydrates, my diet permitted ample fats and animal proteins. This decision flew in the face of the famous diets that had been developed specifically for people with heart problems, like Pritikin and Ornish. For a cardiologist, this was skating on thin ice. But my experience with patients showed that those so-called heart-healthy diets were nearly impossible to stick to, because they relied too heavily on the dieters' ability to eat superlow fat over the long haul. The South Beach diet would permit lean beef, pork, veal, and lamb.

The low-fat regime's severe restrictions on meat were unnecessary — the latest studies had showed that lean meat did not have a harmful effect on blood chemistry. Even egg yolks are good for you — they're a source of natural vitamin E and have a neutral-to-favourable effect on our balance between good and bad cholesterol, contrary to what we once believed. Chicken, turkey, and fish (especially the oily ones such as salmon, tuna, and mackerel) were recommended on my diet, along with nuts and low-fat cheeses and yogurt. As a rule, low-fat prepared foods *can* be a bad idea — the fats are replaced with carbs, which are themselves fattening. But dairy products such as cheese, milk, and yogurt that are low fat are exceptions to this rule — they are nutritious and not fattening.

I also allowed plenty of healthy mono- and polyunsaturated fats, like the Mediterranean ones: olive oil, rapeseed oil, and peanut oil. These are the good fats. They can actually reduce the risk of heart attack or stroke. In addition to being beneficial, they taste good and make food palatable. They're filling, too — a major consideration for a diet that promises you won't have to go hungry.

Next, I found a suitable guinea pig for preliminary testing purposes, a middle-aged man who was having trouble keeping his growing paunch under control: me. I went on the diet. I gave up bread, pasta, rice, potatoes. No beer. No fruit even, at least in the very beginning, because it contains high levels of fructose, or fruit sugar. But otherwise I was determined to eat as normally as possible, meaning three meals a day plus snacks when I was hungry.

After just a week, I noticed a difference. I lost almost 8 pounds in those first seven days, and it was easy. I didn't suffer any hunger pangs. No terrible cravings. No noticeable deprivation.

Almost sheepishly, I approached Marie Almon, MSRD, chief clinical dietitian at our hospital, Mount Sinai Medical Center in Miami Beach, and told her of my experiment. She conceded that the low-fat diet we had been recommending to cardiac patients wasn't working. So we took the basic principles I had developed and expanded them into an agreeable eating plan.

Practical solutions

We settled on a few more guidelines, based on my clinical experience and study of the literature. First, we acknowledged the primary failing of diets we had tried with patients: They're too complicated and too rigid. A diet may be medically or nutritionally sound, but if it is hard to live with, if it doesn't take into account how human beings operate – the whole person, not just his or her digestive tract and metabolism – then it is a failure. So this diet would be flexible and simple, with as few rules as possible. It would allow people to eat the way people actually *like* to eat, while improving their blood chemistry and helping them lose weight and maintain the loss over the long run. This means a lifetime, not three months or a year. Only by accomplishing these goals would this pro-gramme make the crucial transition from being a diet to being a lifestyle – a way of living and eating that normal human beings can sustain for the rest of their lives.

With that in mind, we decided that we wouldn't ask people to deny themselves every eating pleasure indefinitely. Typically, once you've gone off track on a diet, once you've strayed, you're on your own – the experts never allow for human frailty or tell you how to accommodate the inevitable slips as part of the plan. As a result, people who cheat a little today usually cheat a little more tomorrow, and then it's a slippery slope down to where the diet's in shambles, you've broken every rule, and you're depressed and discouraged and back at square one. So we make ample use of desserts devised especially by Marie Almon for the programme. These treats are delicious, yet use only 'legal' ingredients.

We also simply recognized that there will be days when you just *need* that chocolate ice-cream or lemon meringue pie. I'm a chocoholic myself, so believe me, I understand. This plan would allow dieters to bend or break the rules, so long as they understand exactly what damage they've done and how to undo it. If the cheating did put a few pounds on, or stall the weight loss, the setback would be minimal and easily repaired, rather than spelling doom. One beauty of the three-phase structure of the South Beach Diet is that you can move easily from one stage to another. If, while in Phase 2, you go on vacation and overindulge in sweets, it's easy to switch back to Phase 1 for a week, lose the weight those desserts put on, and then return to where you left off in Phase 2.

Finally, people are practical beings. Diets that require complex menus, or supplements taken at certain times of day, or foods eaten in precise combinations, are just too burdensome to sustain for long. Many popular diets are extremely tricky in that regard, despite the fact that there is no basis in science for such complexity. And so they fail. Most of us lead complicated enough lives without having to be within walking distance of a refrigerator every two hours. Nobody wants to carry around a pillbox or a rule book (or both). So this diet would be based on dishes that are easy to make, with ingredients that are commonly found in supermarkets or even most restaurants. The plan requires snacks between meals, but the kind that can be thrown into a briefcase or backpack in the morning and eaten on the run. Our diet is also distinguished by the absence of calorie counts; percentage counts of fats, carbs, and proteins; or even rules about portion size. Our major concern is that dieters eat good carbs and good fats. Once that's all under control, portions and percentages take care of themselves. By choosing the right carbs and the right fats, you simply won't be hungry all the time.

Our diet, we decided, would have to be effective regardless of the dieter's exercise habits. Without a doubt, exercise does increase the body's metabolism, thereby making the diet more efficient. It is also a critical part of any cardiac health plan. However, the South Beach Diet does not depend on exercise in order to work. You'll lose more weight, faster, if you are active on a regular basis. But you'll lose weight even if you're not.

Flexibility and common sense, guided by real science – as opposed to the pop science that often passes for nutrition these days – were the guiding principles of the South Beach Diet. We hoped we had come up with a workable, practical solution to the obesity that plagued so many people we saw in the hospital setting. We believed it would work for most of them. But of course, we wouldn't really know until they tried it.

MY SOUTH BEACH DIET

KAREN G.:

I'VE LOST 2 STONE 2 LB AND KEPT IT OFF.

I had just moved back to Miami Beach from Arizona after getting a divorce. And, of course, everybody in that situation goes on what I call the Divorce Diet – you know, you're going to be dating people for the first time in a long, long time. And those 30 extra pounds you put on during 30 years of marriage? Back when you thought it didn't matter?

Anyway, I read about the South Beach Diet in the newspaper and it sounded easy, so I got all the details. My big thing is that I hate feeling hungry. I just don't like the sensation. In the past, I had been on plenty of low-fat diets, and I *always* felt hungry. On this diet, though, the rule is that if you feel hungry, you eat. When you sit down to a meal, you're supposed to eat until you're satisfied.

Salty and starchy things were always my weakness, much more than sweets – crisps, chips, popcorn. I would go to a supermarket and the first thing I bought was a large bag of popcorn, and by the time I was through shopping it was finished. And I never went to a movie without having buttered popcorn – never, ever, ever. I had a husband who wanted dinner from soup to nuts, every night: Salad, meat, potatoes, a vegetable, bread – always bread. For me to sit down in a restaurant and not have bread and butter was a big sacrifice. You know, on most diets they say you can have the bread but not the butter. On this diet you can have the butter, but not the bread. Or if you have the bread, it's whole grain dipped in olive oil instead of slathered with butter.

It wasn't so easy for me in the first few weeks, during the strict phase. I had to cut out all the things I loved – bread, potatoes, rice, pasta, crisps. I actually didn't feel so great. I felt… not bad, exactly, but not completely myself either. For the first three weeks I felt like I was getting all that bad stuff out of my system. And while I never was hungry, I still craved all the things I couldn't have.

I don't even have the desire for them now, though. The cravings went away. Now when I want a salad I can have it – and with dressing on it. *Real* dressing, not some crappy stuff that tastes horrible.

My mother went on the diet when she saw the weight I lost. She's 81 and she's got terrible cholesterol, too. After the first couple of weeks she said, 'You know, I'm feeling hungry.' And I said to her, 'Mom, the point of this diet is that you don't *have* to be hungry. *Eat.* If you're hungry, go get a piece of cheese.' She had assumed that if it's a diet, you're supposed to be hungry. She took my advice and started eating, and she still lost about a stone, which she had never been able to take off before.

I'm pretty born again about this diet. I don't cheat a lot. No pasta at all. No rice at all. I can have brown rice, but I don't like it. No potatoes, except for sweet potatoes, and even then, only baked. And not so often. No sweets. I *have* added bread back, because I still love it. Not every day – maybe two or three times a week. And never white. I'll have wholemeal, or rye, or pumpernickel, but even then I always ask if there's any white flour in it. Because many times, there *is*. Rye bread you buy at the supermarket has white flour in it, for instance. So you have to watch it.

Honestly, the best part about this programme is that there isn't a restaurant I can't go into. For lunch, just about any restaurant can make you a salad with vegetables and cheese or meat or fish in it. You can get chicken salad or tuna salad anywhere, too. I can go to Burger King and get a barbecued chicken sandwich and throw away the bread. I go to an Italian restaurant that fixes me veal parmigiana without the coating – just tomato sauce and cheese on top. We'll go to a steak house and I'll have prawn cocktail and steak with a vegetable – steamed asparagus or green beans, and I can put butter on it, too. I don't overdo it, but it's real butter. And I'll have a salad with blue cheese dressing. And that's not cheating!

I went on the diet three years ago and I've lost 2 stone 2 lb and kept it off. I feel comfortable again. I'm a size 14 now, and I feel fine the way I am. I would love to lose another 10 pounds, but I'm not going to kill myself to do it. I *was* wearing a size 18. So I had to go to the fat-lady store. It's not fun to go to the fat-lady store.

a day in the life

I started this book by describing, in a nutshell, how you would pass the initial weeks on the South Beach Diet. Now I'll back up and tell you in greater detail how a typical day will go.

Let's start with the first day of Phase 1. You no doubt treated yourself to a memorable meal the night before, but whatever carb-driven cravings you prompted came as you slept, with no further damage done. By the time you wake up today, your bloodstream is a relatively clean slate. The immediate goal is to *keep* it that way. We will accomplish that simply by not introducing any bad carbs into your system.

We'll begin with a two-egg omelette fortified by two slices of lean bacon, cooked in a spray of olive or rapeseed oil. You may yearn for your usual toast or bagel, but if you can get your mind off bread, the rest of you will follow. This will be your first test of the new regime. It may take a few days to wean yourself from the customary morning dose of carbs. But it's our goal in Phase 1 to begin reversing your body's likely inability to process sugars and starches properly, the condition at the root of most weight problems. To accomplish this, we need to cut off all carbs but the healthiest ones, meaning we'll have those highest in fibre and nutrients and lowest in sugars and starches – vegetables and salads only, in other words, at least for these two weeks.

This morning's combination of proteins (the eggs and lean bacon) and good fats (the oil and the bacon), will keep your stomach full and occupied with digestion. You won't have to contend with hunger pangs now or later this morning. It didn't have to be the bacon omelette – we could have gone with two eggs and some asparagus, broccoli, mushrooms, or peppers. That would have introduced some good vegetable fibre to the mix. An omelette with ham or low-fat cheese would have been fine too.

With this meal you can have coffee or tea if you like, with low-fat milk and sugar substitute. There are many sugar substitutes to choose from nowadays – I prefer one that's actually derived in part from a form of sugar, although it has no calories. Some diets prohibit coffee or tea because caffeine does intensify cravings somewhat. But you've got enough changes to contend with without having to give up your morning coffee too.

A phenomenon I've noticed when dealing with overweight people is how many of them skip breakfast altogether. Especially women, for some strange reason. It's not even necessarily an attempt to save on calories – they say they just don't like eating first thing in the morning. The problem is that this allows blood sugar to drop and hunger to increase over the course of the morning, resulting in powerful cravings for a lunch that includes carbs of questionable value – the very kind guaranteed to keep you overweight. So, especially if you're trying to fight off obesity, skipping breakfast is a bad idea.

Planning your meals

In Part II, we've provided a meal by meal, dish by dish eating plan for every phase of the diet. As you'll see, the array of breakfasts even in the strict first phase is varied. There's a frittata made with smoked salmon, for instance, and something we call Vegetable Quiche Cups To Go, which are made with eggs and spinach and, for the sake of convenience, can be prepared in advance and then microwaved at mealtime. We make liberal use of eggs for breakfast, which will alarm some people who have been taught to avoid them due to cholesterol concerns. It turns out that eggs contain no saturated fat and raise the good cholesterol along with the bad. The yolk is a good source of natural vitamin E and protein too. So up to seven eggs a week are permissible. By the second phase of the diet, we'll begin to reintroduce carbs, even toast and muffins, along with some cereals. Fruit, too.

Whether you feel the need for a mid-morning snack or not, you should be ready for one by 10.30 or so. Wisely, you remembered to pack a chunk of low-fat cheese. As I said in chapter two, the only low-fat foods I recommend for dieters are cheese and yogurt, because they're the only ones that don't add bad carbs to replace the fats. The sugar is limited to lactose – milk sugar – which is an acceptable component of the South Beach Diet. Not low-fat ones! They're convenient and they taste good. Most important, they do the job of filling you up with good fats and proteins. That means you won't arrive at the lunch hour feeling famished.

When lunch rolls around, you may have a salad – lettuce and tomato mixed with grilled chicken or fish, dressed in a vinaigrette made with olive oil. You'll also have water or a beverage containing no sugar. Another day you might choose grilled prawn on a bed of green salad, or a tomato stuffed with tuna salad. Niçoise salad is great, too. All these dishes can easily be made at home and, thanks to the trend towards fresh, healthy dining out, can usually be found in restaurants, too. Don't even think about limiting the amount you eat – the point of this diet is to eat well. Food is one of life's dependable pleasures, and it can be a wholesome one if you're eating the proper things. Accomplish that and you will be free to indulge in the improper things from time to time.

I hope you are beginning to see the pattern of these meals: They're all combinations of healthy carbohydrates, proteins, and fats. They are normal, everyday dishes intended to fully satisfy your hunger while depriving your system of the low-quality sugars and starches that have wreaked such havoc on your blood chemistry. You may have noticed that we're not discussing calorie counts, fat grams, or portion sizes. The South Beach Diet is designed so that you don't pay attention to any of that. One hallmark of this programme is its simplicity – life is complicated enough without having to analyse your food before you eat it. If you're eating the right foods you don't need to be obsessive over how much of them you eat. Since fats create the sensation of satiety much more efficiently than carbs do, you won't sit in front of the TV all night popping bites of steak into your mouth, though you can easily imagine snacking for hours on crisps or biscuits!

By the time you finish this book, you'll have a strong overall grasp of which foods you can eat freely, which you need to enjoy in moderation, and which you'll do without. You'll understand the principles of metabolism – not as a matter of academic interest but in a practical, nuts-and-bolts way that will give you a basic understanding of how foods affect your blood chemistry and how that then determines what you weigh. You'll actually learn how to control your blood chemistry and your metabolism through food choices.

Knowing how individual foods affect your internal workings will help you lose weight and maintain the loss. In the future, if you ease up on the diet and find you've gained a few pounds, you'll know how to undo the damage. The glycemic indexes of foods, which are explained and identified on pages 29–33, will be important tools to help you understand which foods contribute to obesity. But once you learn the basics, you'll have all the knowledge you'll need to eat properly. You'll find it easy to cook at home or eat out while sticking to the plan.

Changing your thinking

Okay, by now it's mid-afternoon, typically the first dangerous time of day, dietwise. This is when you might normally crave a sugar fix, owing to the natural dip in blood sugar and consequently, energy, that takes place about this time. This is when people tend to run to the coffee shop, the sweet counter, or the vending machines. Instead, you'll have nuts – let's say plain almonds (not salted or smoked). Nuts contain good, healthy fats, and they fill you up. It's possible to have too many of them, however, and undermine your weight loss. I recommend counting out 15 almonds or cashews or whatever you choose. Some people have told me they prefer pistachios, in part because they're so small that you can allow yourself 30 of them. Cracking and eating 30 pistachios makes it a more elaborate, and therefore more satisfying, snack.

Now it's time to begin thinking about dinner. Recent trends in fine food have brought us all towards something close to the South Beach Diet way of thinking – fresh vegetables, fish, and lean meats are the staples of dinner on our programme. So Phase I features dishes such as grilled salmon with lemon, roasted aubergine and a salad, chicken made with balsamic vinegar, or even marinated rump steak and mushroom caps stuffed with spinach. You could happen upon any of these on the menu of a good restaurant and be happy with them. And this is the *strict* phase of the diet! As you'll see in Part II, in the meal plans for Phase I, we rely on chicken, fish, lean beef, and plenty of vegetables and salads to go with them.

We strongly recommend that you have dessert after that meal. The second dangerous time of day is between dinner and bedtime. This is when all good intentions and strong resolve are challenged. Partly it's just the normal nightly routine – you unwind with a book or in front of the TV, perhaps in the company of friends or family, and the communal snacking habit kicks in. If you've got children, as I do, you've almost certainly got lots of temptations around the kitchen. Or it may just be that you've trained yourself to expect something sweet after a savoury dinner.

In any event, we've come up with two basic strategies for dessert during Phase 1. The first, and simplest, is to have some sugar-free gelatine. For people who love fruit, it may even make up for the loss of fresh fruit flavours during these two weeks. The other suggestion makes ample use of low-rat ricotta cheese. You can use it as the basis for a number of delicious, permissible desserts. This one is reminiscent of the Italian delicacy known as tiramisu, which combines cheese, chocolate, espresso, and ladyfingers: Instead, you take 110g (4 oz) of low-fat ricotta and stir in a few teaspoons of unsweetened cocoa powder, some slivered almonds, and a sachet of sugar substitute. It tastes great, and I guarantee that when you're done you'll feel as though you've had a real dessert. We've tried a number of variations on this – using vanilla or almond extract, lemon zest, or even topping the ricotta with sugar-free chocolate syrup and then baking it.

And that's day one of the South Beach Diet! By the time you finish the last bite of mocha ricotta, you will have already begun ridding your being of the cravings that pushed you into the growing (in every way) ranks of the overweight. Your blood is different from the way it was 24 hours ago: Healthier. Get through another day this way and you'll be even closer to your goal of weight loss, and my goal for you, of better overall health.

MY SOUTH BEACH DIET

DANIEL S.:

I FOUND THIS DIET EXTREMELY EASY.

I went to my doctor and said I needed a diet. And I said, 'I don't want you to give me pills.' I'm six-one and I weighed 19 stone. In my early twenties I was even heavier – probably close to 21 stone. I lost some of that, but then yo-yoed around with the rest. Physically, I'm in very good shape. Cholesterol, blood pressure, heart – fine. But I was feeling lethargic – unable to move around the way I should.

I go out to dinner a lot. And I was just loading up on a lot of bad things.

I am definitely a stress eater, so there were a lot of potatoes and pasta and stuff like that at night. Bread – I soaked it up.

For breakfast, I was always good. Lunch, I tended to be pretty good. It was late afternoon – snack-time – into dinner that was the problem. My afternoon pick-me-up would be a chocolate bar or biscuits or something. Clearly not what I should be eating.

And then for dinner – whatever I wanted. I put no limits on myself. Dessert included.

I would say that my downfall was starchy foods. 4 to 8 p.m. was the bad zone. An extreme day – a stressful day – would be different starting in the morning. I might have doughnuts or some kind of cake. I'd get an attitude that says: Hey – life's stressful. Might as well enjoy what you can.

I've been on this diet around a year and two months now. As I said, I've gone on a hundred diets before this one. A million diets. I've gone from very good results to just moderate. It's very easy for me to lose weight. It's been nearly impossible for me to keep it off. I'd lose for four months, six months. And then it would creep back up.

I found this diet extremely easy. I could reintroduce a lot of stuff into my eating after the initial strict phase of the diet. I found that, as we added foods back, I was able to live a fairly normal life, with some modifications of my own. The main thing is teaching myself that, after lunchtime, I cannot put bread, potatoes, or pasta into my system. So that's how I've lived the past year, not eating any of those foods after, say, 5 p.m. I can live without pasta and potatoes. But bread is the one I'm still weak for. And so I've just forced myself to do without it. At a restaurant I ask the waiter not to bring bread to the table. That's not to say I haven't had bread in the last year. But when I have had it – or potatoes or pasta – at night, it shows up as a stall in my weight loss. So there's a clear correlation between those three items and maintaining my weight.

On certain occasions – my birthday, for one, a few weeks ago – I went to a great Italian restaurant, and they made homemade pasta. I had a bowl and I soaked it up with garlic bread. It was phenomenal. But it was my birthday. I should enjoy myself on my birthday. I also had dessert that night. But the next night, and ever since that night, I haven't had any of that stuff.

For lunch or breakfast I'll have a little bread sometimes. Never later than that. And I don't feel denied at all. That's the difference between now and the past. There are times where I see bread and think: Oh, gee, I'd really love a piece. But I've taught myself to go without it.

how eating makes you hungry

How eating makes you *what*?

Weren't you always under the impression that eating is what *satisfies* hunger?

Well, it is and it isn't. Eating does put an immediate end to hunger. But some foods also create new cravings by making you hungrier than you would be if you hadn't eaten them.

This isn't just a theory, or a matter of perception.

Dr David S. Ludwig is the head of the obesity programme at Children's Hospital in Boston, a physician who also teaches at Harvard Medical School. He is doing some of the medical world's most important research into the root causes of our weight problems. Ludwig recently studied how the breakfast eaten by some obese teenagers influenced their hunger levels hours later.

Three groups of overweight adolescents were fed breakfasts of identical calorie counts. One group's meal was 20 percent fat, 16 percent protein, and roughly two-thirds carbs, but the good kind — steel-cut porridge oats, meaning the flakes were large and the kernel of the oat was unprocessed, and so the fibre was intact. The second group also had a two-thirds-carbs breakfast, but they were served *instant* porridge, where the fibre has been stripped away to permit shorter cooking time.

The third group's meal was identical to a typical South Beach Diet breakfast — vegetable omelettes.

After breakfast, members of all three groups were instructed to eat anything they wanted for the next five hours.

The subjects who had the bad carb breakfast – the instant porridge group – ate the most during that five-hour period. They also reported feeling the strongest hunger pangs.

The teenagers who had the steel-cut porridge oats felt less hunger and ate less than the instant porridge group during the post-breakfast hours.

The group who had the vegetable omelettes – the low-carb meal – reported the lowest sensation of hunger and ate the smallest amount during the five hours after breakfast.

This is one of several recent studies testing the theory that eating bad carbs makes you hungrier, and that on a diet of good carbs and good fats (the vegetable omelette combines both) you'll want less food later. I'll explain exactly why this happens, but for now I want to emphasize what all the studies show: Eating bad carbohydrates – especially highly processed ones – creates cravings for more bad carbs, which ultimately is responsible for our epidemic of obesity. It's hard to overstate the connection between bad carbs and bad nutritional and cardiac health.

In another diet and hunger study, subjects who ate whole fruit reported less hunger than those who ate purée of the same fruit, and those who ate purée had fewer cravings than those who just drank the juice. In various other research projects, scientists found that eating beans causes less hunger than eating potatoes; raw carrots cause less hunger than cooked ones; foods containing whole grains cause less hunger than those containing cracked grains; ordinary rice causes less hunger than the instant variety.

There's a term for the basic physiological response to food that's behind all these findings: reactive hypoglycemia.

I will describe exactly what that means. But before I tell you, let me show you.

For years, every day at around 3 or 4 in the afternoon, I'd find myself running out of steam – weak, sleepy, sometimes even light-headed. Without thinking, I'd make a run for the doctors' lounge, where I would ingest a bran muffin and a cup of coffee. I actually thought that since the muffin was labelled low fat, it was healthy. In fact, the word *bran* was there mainly to keep people from examining the ingredients closely and realizing that the muffin was just a fairy cake in disguise. Even physicians were lulled into a false sense of security – the fat in the muffin may have been low, but the carbs it contained contributed quite a bit of fat to my waistline.

Having finished my snack, I instantly felt better. So give my body credit for knowing exactly what it needed: Carbs. *Sugar*. My body knew this because it detected that the level of glucose – the form sugar takes in our bloodstreams – had fallen too low. Glucose is a form of chemical energy that our brains in particular need on a constant basis in order to function properly. Without enough, we'd grow dizzy, faint, and eventually go into a coma and die. Diabetes is the body's inability to turn food into usable forms of energy; this is why without synthetic insulin, type I diabetics would not live for long.

So my brain detects hypoglycemia – too-low blood sugar – and my body reacts (hence the name reactive hypoglycemia) by creating the cravings that drove me, and maybe you, too, towards the nearest carbohydrate fix.

How carbs work

As we've already said, carbohydrates are contained in a vast and varied array of foods, everything from the most virtuous vegetable to the most decadent treat. All carbs contain sugars. These sugars, though, exist in several different forms and go by a variety of names, including maltose (in beer), sucrose (table sugar), lactose (in dairy), and fructose (as found in fruit).

Despite that similarity, no one who has ever craved a sugar doughnut has been satisfied by broccoli. The opposite might also be true, though it's difficult to find people who suffer from insatiable cravings for green vegetables.

It's easy to tell by taste which carbs are highest in sugars, and which yield their sugars most readily. It probably comes as no surprise that a milk chocolate bar gives up its sugars more freely than one made of dark chocolate, or a pineapple yields its sweetness faster than a grapefruit, or a slice of supermarket white bread produces blood sugar faster than a piece of Ryvita. The more sugar there is, and the faster it's released, the more acutely we sense that sugar 'rush' – the relief that courses through our bloodstream as we heed the call for carbs. Internally, though, our bodies treat all carbs in basically the same way – digestion is in large part the process by which our bodies extract the sugars from carbohydrates and turn them into fuel, which we either burn or store. Burning the fuel is good – that means we're active enough to make efficient use of the food we eat. Storage of a little fuel is all right, but anything more than that is not so good. You know that excess stored fuel by another term: body fat.

The job of carbohydrate digestion starts in our mouths, when we chew the food into bits and our saliva begins the chemical process of separating each mouthful into its components. In our stomachs, the food is further shredded by the organ's muscular contractions and gastric acids. Our bodies want to get at the sugars contained in carbs, but this happens at varying speeds, depending on certain factors. Essentially, the less encumbered these sugars are by other substances, the faster they enter our bloodstreams.

Carbs' competitors

Which substances get in our bodies' way? Fibre is the major factor that slows the absorption of sugar. That's the reason the highly processed oatmeal was worse, diet-wise, than the steel-cut variety – the latter had all the fibre still intact, and so before the stomach could get to the sugars in the oatmeal, it had to separate them from the fibre. Once isolated, the fibre passes undigested through your system; its dietary importance comes from its ability to slow digestion down. It's an obstacle to digestion – a good one.

This was demonstrated not long ago in a scientific study in which half the subjects were given the fibre known as psyllium (you probably know it better as Fybogel) 15 minutes before lunch. The other half had lunch without the psyllium first. In the hours after the meal, the fibre group reported less hunger than the others. As the day wore on they ate less, too. The reason is simple: In their stomachs, the psyllium mixed in with what they ate and drank and slowed down the digestion. Slower digestion of carbs, less insulin. Less insulin, less dramatic drop in blood sugar. Less of a sugar rise and fall now, less hunger later.

Fibre isn't the only thing that slows the digestion of carbohydrates. Fat, too, slows the speed at which your stomach accesses the sugars you've eaten. That's why, in the study of overweight adolescents, the omelette breakfast created the least desire to eat more later. We have found other factors that slow the digestion of carbs and therefore benefit dieters. Acidic foods such as lemon and vinegar slow the speed with which your stomach empties, therefore cutting back on the rise in blood sugar. You can dress salads or vegetables in both and enjoy the benefit. Even sourdough bread, while not high in fibre, is acidic, and will improve any meal.

This is an important lesson in eating properly and losing weight on the South Beach Diet. This is why we call carbs containing fibre *good*, and why we also think of certain fats as good, too: Anything that slows the process by which you process the sugars in carbs is, by definition, good.

The body's response

Once the food has been liquefied in the stomach, it travels downwards to our small intestine, where millions of capillaries absorb what we've eaten and transport it into our bloodstream. Once there, it travels through our liver and then everywhere else in our bodies to be used, stored, or eliminated.

But let's continue to focus on the carbs. As we've said, they all contain sugar in one form or another. Even the starches are merely chains of sugars; digestion cuts the links in order to make the sugar molecules available to us. What we're concerned with here is the *speed* with which our bodies get at the sugars. It doesn't all take place at the same rate.

Once the sugars enter our bloodstream, it is the job of the pancreas to detect this and go to work – producing the hormone insulin in sufficient quantity to get the sugars out of our blood and into the organs where it is needed, or into storage for future needs. This is where diabetics run into trouble: They ingest the same sugars as everyone else, but without effective insulin those sugars remain uselessly circulating in the bloodstream. Insulin unlocks our tissues and lets the sugars in.

Fortunately, the pancreas can tell how much insulin is needed to do that job. If the body experiences a fast infusion of sugars, a lot of insulin is required. If the sugars are metabolized more slowly, the insulin is released gradually.

This is a crucial difference, as far as obesity is concerned: Fast sugar is worse for you; slower is better.

Here's why. When the sugars are absorbed slowly, the rise in blood sugar is gradual and so, too, is its descent once the insulin begins to do its work. The slow decline in blood sugar translates into less insistent cravings for more carbs later. You recall what I described as reactive hypoglycemia – the sensation of hunger caused by low blood sugar.

When the decline in blood sugar is gentle, the cravings are lessened.

But when your pancreas detects a rapid rise in blood sugar, it pumps out a correspondingly high level of insulin to do the job. That results in a rapid plunge in the blood sugar level. The insulin ends up doing its job a little too well – the blood sugar level drops so low that new cravings are created, requiring more quick carbohydrate fixes. In order to satisfy so many cravings, of course, we take in well beyond the nutrition we require. We overeat, and this leads to more fat, more insulin resistance, more hunger, and more weight gain – a vicious cycle.

Therefore, we can most easily stop ourselves from overeating by two strategies:

1. We can eat the foods (and combinations of foods) that cause gradual rather than sharp increases and decreases in blood sugar.

2. We can learn to anticipate hypoglycemia and avert it with the timely consumption of snacks. This one is crucial: It takes much less food to prevent hypoglycemia than it does to resolve it.

The third thing we all should do is learn which foods cause the most rapid rise in blood sugar. In the early 1980s, Dr David Jenkins led a team of Canadian researchers who devised a scale to measure the rapidity and degree with which a fixed quantity of a food increases your blood sugar. They called it the glycemic index. It lists most carbohydrates, from table sugar, beer, and white bread at one extreme to spinach and lentils at the other. On pages 29–33 you will find a sample of the index, organized by food type. You probably won't be completely surprised by what you find there. Anything made with white flour is high on the list. That includes most desserts, breads, and baked goods, of course, but also pasta. Instant rice is also near the top. Certain tropical fruits are fairly high, as are some starchy vegetables, particularly potatoes and other root vegetables. The king of all sugars, the one that increases blood sugar faster than any other, is maltose, which exists in beer. Now you understand what's behind the beer belly: The rapid rise of blood sugar caused by guzzling this beverage stimulates a corresponding rise in insulin production, which encourages storage of fat around the mid-section.

Knowledge and use of the glycemic index of foods is becoming widespread, but there's an important caveat which is crucial to understanding the link between carbs and obesity. You must bear in mind that the degree to which your blood sugar is raised depends not just on the glycemic index of the food but also on the quantity. For example, carrots have a high glycemic index, but they are fairly low in carbohydrate density. Therefore, you'd have to eat several handfuls of carrots to approximate the total rise in blood sugar you'd get from a single slice of white bread.

I have a handy analogy I use to explain this concept to my patients.

Think of alcohol. When we drink it, our blood alcohol level rises, and when it goes above a certain threshold, we feel tipsy. When it rises further, we feel drunk. We know that when we drink on an empty stomach, we get drunk faster. If, on the other hand, we drink while eating, on a full stomach, it takes more alcohol for us to feel the effect. This is because when the drinks mix with the food in our stomach, it takes longer for our bodies to get at and absorb the alcohol into our bloodstream, which transports it to our brain, creating that intoxicated sensation. The principle at work here is this: The more slowly the alcohol is absorbed, the less it affects us.

Now let's consider what happens when we eat carbs – bread, for instance.

If we eat white bread, we're getting no fibre with our carbs. That's like drinking on an empty stomach: Our stomachs can get at the starches without having to first separate them from the fibre. As a result, the bread is quickly turned into glucose – blood sugar – and causes an equally sharp rise in insulin, which brings about the dreaded acute rise and fall of blood sugar level, thereby creating more cravings later on. Eating white bread is analogous to drinking alcohol on an empty stomach; eating whole grain bread is like eating with your cocktail.

The fibre is the part of the grain not absorbed into the bloodstream from the intestine but excreted as waste. Even though it is not absorbed, fibre helps digestion in another, more commonly understood way. It helps your colon to function efficiently – the lack of fibre in our diets is why constipation has become a common problem.

Fibre, then, joins fat, protein, and acidity on the list of things that delay the absorption of sugars and starches. We need to include one or more of the above in every meal in order to keep ourselves from getting drunk – on carbs. By choosing the right foods, food combinations, and strategically timed snacks, you can prevent hypoglycemia and thereby control your weight without having to fight off cravings.

A final anecdote to illustrate this principle: A friend and patient who was in the first week of the diet rushed out one afternoon to play golf. He had neglected to plan his lunch so he decided to break the rules and grab a sandwich. As he played golf, several hours later, he began to feel weak and shaky and recognized this as reactive hypoglycemia. There were no permissible snacks available, so he found some sachets of sugar and guzzled them down. They relieved his acute hunger and they tasted great, too. He returned home and downed a bag of tortilla chips and a chocolate bar. This binge was due not to a loss of self-control but to his poor planning. Once the hypoglycemia struck, the consequence was preordained. Had my friend eaten tuna salad instead of a sandwich and had some low-fat cheese or nuts as a snack, both the initial hypoglycemia and subsequent gorging could have been avoided.

MY SOUTH BEACH DIET:

PAUL L.:

I'VE CLEANED OUT MY MEDICINE CABINET THANKS TO THIS DIET.

I weighed 16½ stone five years ago, when I went on this diet. Over the years, I had always struggled with my weight, and I tried lots of the diets out there. I tried Atkins – in fact, I had actually been a patient of his years ago, before he got famous. And so I tried his low-carb diet. I also tried some of the low-fat diets, the Heart Association-type programmes. I always lost some weight but I always gained it back.

I'm 73 now, and I was 68 when I started with the South Beach Diet. I had been a heavy smoker and then I gave it up, which is how I happened to put on all that weight. I wasn't a big sweets eater. But I loved all the rest. Bread three times a day, with every meal. And potatoes. Rice. Pasta. Of course, meat and so on – big, heavy meals. Once my weight hit its peak, I started getting some other problems, too. One day we found that I had diabetes. My blood pressure was high. My triglycerides were high. My cholesterol was high.

I began seeing Dr Agatston as my cardiologist, and we discussed how my being so overweight was contributing to my conditions. He suggested the diet he developed. And because I was no stranger to diets, I said I'd give it a try.

The first few days weren't exactly easy. I wouldn't say you feel bad, but definitely different. A little off. You're hungry because you're not following your normal eating patterns. But after those first 3 days, it suddenly seemed easier. I wasn't really going hungry. I ate a ton of vegetables during that strict phase, and a lot of meat and fish and cheese, too. A lot of white meat chicken and turkey. But no bread or pasta or even fruit.

After the first two weeks, I started adding things back into my diet. I had some fruit, although to be honest, when I had a little fruit I wanted more. It was easier in a way to just go without fruit altogether.

I never did add any potatoes back to my diet — I just didn't miss them enough to want them, I guess. And maybe it's easier for me to have none than a little. I do like pasta, and so I'll have that every once in a while — say, every few weeks I'll have a dish. Rice, less so, though I'll have that occasionally, too. I have gone back to eating bread. I'll have it just about every day now, and two or three pieces. And I drink red wine — two glasses a day.

It took me about a year, but I went from 16½ down to 12 stone on this diet. 4½ stone in 50 weeks. And for the past four years I've been maintaining this weight pretty easily. Once it crept up again, to 12½, so I just went back on the Phase 1 diet and I got back down to 12 pretty fast.

The best part, though, is that I've cleaned out my medicine cabinet thanks to this diet. I stopped taking the diabetes medicine because it cleared up. Blood pressure medicine — gone. I was taking a statin for my cholesterol, but now I've even thrown that away.

THE GLYCEMIC INDEX

The following table lists the glycemic index of many of the foods you're likely to encounter in your daily life. The choices are grouped by type of food, then arranged alphabetically.

A food's glycemic index is the amount that it increases your blood sugar level compared to the amount that the same quantity of white bread would increase it.

The foods with the lower numbers will cause your blood sugar to rise then fall more slowly that the foods with higher numbers will. Numerous studies have also shown that low-glycemic foods satisfy your hunger longer and minimize your food cravings better.

In Phase 1 of the South Beach Diet, you should only choose foods with a low glycemic index. Later on, after you've gone through the rapid weight-loss phase, you can start mixing in foods with higher numbers.

However, still follow the other rules of the diet; even though skimmed milk and peanut M&Ms have the same glycemic index, the milk is a much better nutritional choice.

BAKERY PRODUCTS	GI
Cake, angel	67
Cake, sponge	46
Cake, tart	65
Croissant	67
Danish pastry	59
Doughnut	76
Muffin (unsweetened sort)	62
Waffles	76

BEVERAGES	GI
Apple juice	41
Carrot juice	45
Grapefruit juice	48
Orange juice	52
Pineapple juice	46
Soya milk	30

BREADS	GI
Bagel, plain	72
Baguette	95
Bread stuffing	74
Hamburger bun	61
Melba toast	70
Multi grain bread	48
Pitta bread, white	57
Pizza, cheese	60
Rye-flour bread	64
Wheat bread, gluten-free	90
White bread	71
White rolls	73
Whole grain e.g. pumpernickel	50
Wholemeal bread	69

BREAKFAST CEREALS	GI
All-Bran	42
Cheerios	74
Cornflakes	83
Golden Grahams	71
Grape-Nuts	67
Mini-Wheats (wholemeal)	57
Muesli	56
Oat bran	55
Porridge, non-instant	49
Puffed Wheat	74
Rice Krispies	82
Shredded Wheat	69
Special K	54
Weetabix	77

CEREAL GRAINS	GI
Barley, cracked	50
Barley flakes	66
Buckwheat flakes	55
Bulgur wheat	48
Couscous	65
Millet	71
Pearl barley	25

Polenta	69
Rice, brown	55
Rice, instant	46
Rice, parboiled	48
Rice, white	58
Rice, wild	57
Rye	34
Taco shells	68
Tapioca, boiled with milk	81
Wheat kernels	41

SWEET BISCUITS — GI

Biscotti	79
Digestives	58
Shortbread	64
Wafer biscuits	77

SAVOURY BISCUITS — GI

Rice cakes	77
Ryvita	67
Water biscuits	65

DAIRY FOODS — GI

Milk, chocolate, artificially sweetened	24
Milk, semi-skimmed	34
Milk, skimmed	32
Milk, whole	27
Ice-cream	61
Ice-cream, low-fat	50
Yogurt, low-fat, artificially sweetened	14
Yogurt, low-fat, fruit-flavoured	33

FRUIT AND FRUIT PRODUCTS — GI

Apples	38
Apricots	57
Apricots, dried	31
Apricots, tinned in syrup	64
Bananas	54
Cherries	22
Fruit cocktail	55
Grapefruit	25
Grapes	46
Kiwi fruit	53
Mangoes	56
Cantaloupe melon	65
Oranges	44
Peaches	42
Peaches, tinned	47
Pears	38
Pears, tinned	44
Pineapple	66
Plums	39
Raisins	64
Watermelon	72

PULSES — GI

Baked beans, tinned	48
Black-eyed beans	41
Broad beans	79
Butter beans, boiled	31
Chickpeas	33
Chickpeas, tinned	42
Haricot beans, boiled	38
Kidney beans, boiled	29
Kidney beans, tinned	52
Lentils, green, boiled	29

Lentils, green, tinned	52		Potato, new	57
Lentils, red, boiled	25		Potato, steamed	65
Lima beans, baby, frozen	32		Potato, tinned	61
Pinto beans	39		Sweet potato	54
Pinto beans, tinned	45		Swede	72
Soya beans, boiled	16		Yam	51
Split peas, yellow, boiled	32			

PASTA	**GI**
Capellini	45
Fettuccine	32
Gnocchi	67
Linguine	46
Macaroni	45
Macaroni cheese	64
Ravioli, meat filled	39
Rice pasta, brown	92
Spaghetti, durum wheat	55
Spaghetti, protein enriched	27
Spaghetti, wholewheat	37
Spaghetti, white	41
Tortellini, cheese	50
Vermicelli	35

ROOT VEGETABLES	**GI**
Beetroot	64
Carrots, cooked	39
Chips	75
Parsnips	97
Potato, baked	85
Potato, boiled	56
Potato, instant	83
Potato, mashed	70
Potato, microwaved	82

SNACK FOOD AND SWEETS	**GI**
Chocolate bar, 30g (1½ oz)	49
Corn chips	74
Crisps	54
Dates	103
Jams and marmalades	49
Jelly beans	80
Life Savers or Refreshers	70
Mars Bar	64
M&Ms (peanut)	32
Skittles	69
Snickers Bar	40
Twix Biscuit Bars (caramel)	43
Peanuts	15
Popcorn	55
Pretzels	81

SOUPS	**GI**
Lentil soup, tinned	44
Tomato soup, tinned	38

SUGARS	**GI**
Fructose powder	22
Honey	58
Lactose	46
Liquid glucose	96

Maltose	105	Kale	<15
Sucrose	64	Lettuce, all varieties	<15
		Mange-tout	<15
VEGETABLES	GI	Mushrooms, all varieties	<15
Artichoke, globe	<15	Mustard greens	<15
Asparagus	<15	Okra	<15
Aubergine	<15	Peanuts	<15
French beans	<15	Peas, dried	22
Green beans	<15	Peas, green	48
Beetroot	<15	Peppers, all varieties	<15
Broccoli	<15	Pumpkin	75
Brussels sprouts	<15	Rocket	<15
Cabbage, all varieties	<15	Spinach	<15
Cauliflower	<15	Spaghetti squash	<15
Celery	<15	Young summer squash	<15
Swiss chard	<15	Sweet corn	55
Courgettes	<15	Tomatoes	15
Cucumber	<15	Turnip	<15
Batavian endive	<15	Watercress	<15

is it diabetes yet?

I see an awful lot of people with the condition largely responsible for the current epidemic of obesity and heart disease. You see them, too, whether you know it or not.

I see them in my examining room, of course, but I also see them on the street, at parties, at the shops, on the beach, virtually everywhere I look. They're very easy to recognize thanks to one unmistakable visible sign: central obesity – excess weight concentrated mainly in a rounded, protruding waistline, often on individuals with the face, arms, and legs you'd expect to find on someone thinner. It's commonly referred to as apple-shaped obesity – as opposed to pear-shaped, where the excess weight is distributed throughout the hips, buttocks, and legs.

People usually refer to central obesity by some cute euphemism – it's a paunch, a beer gut, a potbelly, a bay window. But to me it's a serious warning of unhealthy blood chemistry today and cardiac trouble ahead. In social settings, I have to restrain myself from urging people I've just met who fit the above profile to call me (or any cardiologist) first thing in the morning to schedule diagnostic blood tests. I've become something of an evangelist on this subject because the disorder is so widespread and dangerous, yet simple to treat using diet, exercise, and medication.

When I ask overweight patients about family medical history, they'll frequently tell me about a parent or grandparent who developed diabetes late in life, often in their seventies or eighties. 'But it was just "chemical" diabetes,' the patient will assure me, using an outdated term. 'He didn't even take insulin for it.' Sometimes they'll refer to it as 'sugar' diabetes, another relic of medical terminology. The patient has no idea that this late-occurring form of the disease in a parent is actually an indication that another, silent but potentially deadly condition is present – one that is setting the stage, internally, for his or her own future heart attack or stroke. The diabetes gene is passed along to all offspring. An early manifestation of the disease is weight gain during middle age – years before blood sugar becomes elevated.

But what does diabetes have to do with a heart attack or stroke? That's the question most people ask. Over the past ten years we have come a long way in understanding the connection. We now know without a doubt that they are linked: About half of all people who have heart attacks are found to be suffering from a condition that goes under several names. Metabolic syndrome is the most popular current term, but it's also been called insulin resistance, or syndrome X. We've known of its existence only since 1989, and we're still learning about it. For our purposes let's refer to it as prediabetes, since that comes closest to calling it what it is – an early stage of the disease. Unchecked, prediabetes today will turn into full-blown type 2 diabetes tomorrow.

By the latest count, somewhere around 47 million Americans – close to one in five – are estimated to have prediabetes. But the percentage of adults with cardiovascular disease who also have this syndrome is much higher; maybe half of my practice shows signs. Here's a list of the criteria, according to the National Cholesterol Education Program.

- High cholesterol
- High ratio of bad cholesterol to good
- High blood pressure
- Central obesity
- High triglycerides

To which I would add:

- Small LDL (bad cholesterol) particles

These are also the conditions that are closely associated with heart attack and stroke. Genetics plays a major role in determining whether you'll have these conditions. But so does improper diet. I'll try not to burden you with too much science as I explain the connection between heart disease and adult-onset diabetes. Trust me: It's important to understand this.

The facts on diabetes

Most people know diabetes as the body's inability to process sugars and starches properly. Your body digests a meal and converts all the carbs into glucose – blood sugar. It then becomes the job of your pancreas to detect this sudden infusion of glucose and, in response, produce the hormone insulin. The insulin is needed to allow your body's various organs – brain, muscles, liver, and so on – to extract the glucose from your bloodstream and either use it at once or store it for future use. The body's need for sugar is constant – without it in sufficient quantities you will become dizzy, faint, go into a coma, and before long, die.

Imagine that each cell in your body has a lock on it, and insulin is the only key that fits. If the cells remain locked, the sugars can't enter, and they remain circulating uselessly in your bloodstream, where they do you no good and cause considerable harm.

But what most people don't realize is that diabetes isn't just about how we process sugars: It's also the inability to properly process the fats we eat.

When we eat fats, whether from flesh, vegetable oils, or dairy products, it is also insulin's job to transport the fatty acids (the basic component of fats) from the bloodstream into the body's tissues, where they belong, to be used immediately for fuel or stored for future use in the form we know as triglycerides.

In fact, diabetes can be seen as the body's inability to manage its fuel supply well. Obesity, too, is just a matter of bad fuel management, due to a combination of genetics and lifestyle. Our bodies are designed to store excess energy (which we call calories) for a very good reason: For most of humanity's existence, securing a steady and sufficient supply of food has been our biggest, most important challenge. Feast or famine prevailed and, to adapt, our bodies would save the energy from today's feast, knowing that tomorrow it would need to burn saved fuel in order to survive. That's why this particular brand of obesity concentrates the fat in the mid-section – it leaves the extremities lithe and muscular, for ease of manual labour and, especially, flight. Advanced civilization has done a great deal to eradicate famine, but at the expense of our waistlines and our cardiovascular systems, which now suffer from the fact that we store fat we no longer need. We'd be better off if our bodies eliminated excess energy as if it were waste, but they don't.

This is exacerbated by the physiology of the fat cell. When we gain weight, we're not creating new fat cells – their number remains constant from childhood. No, what happens is that the fat cells themselves get fat. That's why in overweight people the insulin has trouble attaching to the fat cells – they've grown too big. As a result, when an overweight person overeats, it's like trying to fill a gas tank that's already at capacity – the excess spills over. In your body, that means the sugars and fats circulate in your blood longer than they should. When your body cannot properly transfer the glucose and fatty acids from your bloodstream into your tissues, it's the beginning of trouble. Left untreated, serious cases of diabetes would be fatal.

But there are *two* types of diabetes, and these differ in important ways.

Juvenile (or type 1) diabetes usually strikes during childhood or adolescence. It's caused by some damage that's been done to the pancreas – possibly by a virus. As a result, the organ produces too little insulin to do the job of getting sugars and fats from the bloodstream into the proper tissues. It's an incurable disease so far and can be treated only by replacing the insulin with daily insulin injections. That's why eating carefully and measuring blood sugar level are so important to a diabetic's well-being and why insulin is such a lifesaving drug.

We don't even have a proper name yet for the other form of this disease; hence its working title: type 2 diabetes. This is also called adult-onset diabetes, because that's when it usually shows up. As we've said, there's no virus to blame, just who we are (genetics) and what we eat. A surprisingly large percentage of us are genetically predisposed to diabetes of this kind. But the predisposition is just that – the *potential* for diabetes – until poor diet and lack of exercise do their damage. We can't control our genes. But if you can keep from making bad food choices, you can prevent this form of diabetes.

Both these diseases go by the same name, but the causes are opposite. Juvenile diabetes is a result of the pancreas's inability to produce insulin. In type 2, your pancreas is fully functional and is actually making *too much* insulin. We discussed this earlier: When you carry excess body fat, you make it difficult for insulin to do its job. So the blood sugar level doesn't lower as quickly as it should, prompting your pancreas to pump out even more insulin in order to unlock your cells and let the glucose in. Your pancreas sends out insulin until finally it overshoots the mark, which is why the blood sugar level goes so low. It's the high level of sugar in the bloodstream and then the rapid plunge (when you finally produce enough insulin) that causes your sharp food cravings. Which in turn causes you to eat more carbs, and so the vicious cycle goes around and around.

All the above is fine and good as an explanation for why obesity makes you overeat, and why eating carbs, rather than satisfying your hunger, makes you hungry for more. But we still haven't answered this question: What do obesity and type 2 diabetes or prediabetes have to do with heart trouble?

Effects on the heart

It starts with that central obesity. Your expanding mid-section is not due to an increase in the *number* of fat cells in there. No, when you're overweight, the number of cells remains more or less constant, but each cell increases in size. In other words, the fat cells themselves grow fat. When these cells expand, the insulin has trouble attaching to them properly and unlocking them. That's why, if you weigh too much, the sugar and fat levels in your bloodstream rise higher than they should. The insulin key takes longer to open the lock.

That in turn brings about several other conditions of the blood, all of which are further symptoms of type 2 diabetes and even prediabetes, signs that can be seen only by a doctor. They're a familiar list if you've been paying attention to health news over the past decade: High blood pressure, high triglycerides, high total cholesterol, high ratio of bad cholesterol to good, and the relatively unknown but critical matter of too-small bad cholesterol particles.

When insulin isn't working properly, it takes longer than it should to store the fat you just ate. Because of that delay, your liver is being flooded with fatty acids. In response to that, the organ emits harmful particles that deposit fat and cholesterol in the blood vessels of your heart. Future blockages, in other words.

So this, then, is the link between obesity and heart disease. The danger isn't the carbs or the sugars in themselves. It's how they affect your body's ability to process fats. Eating too many jam doughnuts may not cause a heart attack. But it can and does create the conditions that will lead to one. Obesity itself doesn't damage your cardiovascular system. It's just the number-one sign of an unhealthy blood profile, which will someday almost certainly curtail your good health, and maybe your life.

Today, alarmingly, we're seeing type 2 diabetes in young adults and even in adolescents. It's not that we're congenitally less healthy than previous generations. But our habits are much worse. Gym memberships and home treadmills are staples of middle-class life, but the truth is that we perform less physical activity than our parents and grandparents did. Maybe their jobs required more exertion, or they enjoyed fewer labour-saving devices. Perhaps they just walked a lot more than we do.

This lack of exercise extends even to the youngest among us. I am distressed by the levels of physical playtime children now get. The selling of school playing-fields for development and cutting PE in favour of more classroom instruction are disasters in the making. Such short-sighted policies may save money today, but at the expense of our children's health in the decades to come.

Even more harmful than decreasing exercise, however, is how food itself has changed. As we delegate more and more of our food preparation to fast-food restaurants and food manufacturers, its quality has deteriorated — not just in its taste but in its fibre and nutrient content. In a sense, food manufacturers have begun the digestion process for us. We did not appreciate until quite recently that processed foods were bad and have contributed to our epidemic of obesity. We endured hunger once; now the plenty we enjoy translates directly into the load on our dinner plates. The fact that half of all restaurant meals come in the form of fast food has only worsened things. Once, the carbs we ate were less processed than they are today. More of our bread was baked at home or in local bakeries, not factories, and was made with whole grains, not flour that had been overly processed and stripped of all fibre. Back then, convenience and speedy preparation weren't the highest ideals food aspired to — we were in less of a rush, and home cooking meant starting with raw ingredients. Rice had more of its fibre intact, and had to be cooked slowly. Potatoes weren't sliced and frozen or powdered and bought in a box. Children's after-school snacks weren't limited to what could be microwaved. More of what we ate had shelf lives measured in days, not months and sometimes years!

We didn't require large infusions of sugar in every meal, starting with our breakfast cereal and continuing at every feeding up to the late-night snack of crisps. We weren't confronted with fast-food restaurants and chocolate-chip biscuit stands and sandwich bars at every street corner.

Even the impulse towards healthy eating brought us closer to this unhealthy state. Next time you visit a supermarket, examine the nutritional information on all the 'low-fat' products: Invariably, you'll find that processed carbs have been added to replace the fats. Or notice how many breads there are labelled 'vitamin-enriched' or 'fortified', which means so much of the natural fibre (which contains the vitamins) has been stripped away that some nutrients had to be added back in!

I realize that I'm describing more than any one patient's eating patterns: It's the general attitude to nutrition that's to blame for what's happening internally to many millions of us. Usually, the serious damage doesn't show up until you're in your fifties or even sixties. But the invisible harm is being done decades earlier, setting the stage for the future catastrophe.

The cure for this, luckily, is the same as the solution to the overweight problem that vexes millions of people who aren't terribly concerned about their cardiac well-being decades from now. It's what I've tried to codify in a sensible, practical, easy to remember and follow eating plan that the rest of this book is devoted to explaining. But as far as I'm concerned, this is the true goal of any great diet. Looking good on the outside is important, I know. But having beautiful, physically fit blood vessels and healthy blood chemistry as a result makes it that much more important.

MY SOUTH BEACH DIET:

JUDY H.:

I WENT FROM A SIZE 34 TO A SIZE 20.

I'm 55. I'm divorced. About a year or so ago, I weighed 27½ stone.

It runs in my family. On my mother's side, all the parents and their oldest child – but only the oldest child, which includes me – are heavy. I was fairly thin most of my younger years. But after I had my son and daughter, I gained weight, and I would yo-yo up and down. I've been on many diets over the years, and I've always been able to lose weight. Once I lost 7 stone on a very strict diet. But I eventually gained it back.

I was never a breakfast person. Wasn't a coffee drinker. I don't smoke, I don't drink. I would eat nothing all morning, not even a snack. And for lunch I would just eat whatever everybody else in my office was having. I didn't put a lot of thought into it. It could be Chinese food, it could be hamburgers. Whatever the girls were ordering. We had a lot of full lunches brought in – pasta was a big thing for me at lunch.

After that I didn't eat again until dinner. No snacks in the afternoon. And then dinner-time was usually meat, a vegetable, a salad, and a starch. Pasta. Or potatoes. I was never a rice person. But I really liked my other carbs – pizza and sandwiches too. I would rather eat a sandwich than sit down and have steak and potatoes. Pastry also – I love pastries. Not a sweet eater, but I liked my breads and desserts. I wasn't a big fizzy drinks fan. I was never really that thirsty – that was another problem.

Everybody said, 'Go to Weight Watchers.' 'Try Jenny Craig.' I've tried everything. One day I was talking to one of the girls in our office and I said to her, 'Hey, you look great.' And she says, 'Oh, I'm on this diet I just heard about, Dr Agatston's diet.' So she gave me a copy. And I just took it and ran with it. And I've lost 9½ stone in the year or so since.

But at first when I looked at this diet and I saw that it restricted carbs, I said, 'I'll never be able to do it.' But then I said, 'Well, you *gotta* do it.' So I decided: There will be no more bread in the house. No more milk in the house. I must have had 20 boxes of pasta in the kitchen. Threw it all out. I told my daughter, 'Look, if you need a sandwich, go buy a roll and make one. I just can't have it lying around here.' I got rid of everything, and I never brought it back into the house.

And, still, to this day, I miss my bread – I really do. I would kill to sit down and eat Italian bread with some butter. But I won't do it. Because I know I can't control myself with that stuff. In the past few weeks I found myself close to slipping a little – like wanting just a taste of this or that. Things I wouldn't even think of tasting before. I asked somebody I know at work, 'Do you notice me doing anything different?' And he said, 'Yes, I do – when we have lunch in the office, before you wouldn't touch one morsel of something that you weren't supposed to have. Now you'll take a spoon or two.' So maybe I've slipped a little. But that's good to know. I'm going to have to watch it with carbs for the rest of my life.

The first day wasn't bad. I felt, like, I *have* to do it. This is my last chance. And I started and just stayed on it. I could see the difference the first week. Within six weeks I lost 3½ stone. After that, I began to incorporate more fruits and vegetables into my diet, and some mayonnaise in my tuna, things like that. But I stayed away from having even a little bit of cereal or porridge. No starches. Now and then, as a treat, I might have allowed myself a little piece of a roll of something. But I stop myself. If I go out, I only go to restaurants where I know I can eat the food. I'm not going to kill myself and sit in an Italian restaurant. I know better. I'll go to a Chinese restaurant if I know they don't use MSG (monosodium glutamate). You can pick out your own fresh meat and vegetables and things and they'll stir-fry them for you. So I go there maybe twice a week. I'm a big seafood person. I'll eat mussels, crab legs, prawns. They have green beans cooked with oil and garlic. I'll eat a whole plate of them. Iced tea with Sweet'n Low or a diet drink. I go home full. That's my treat, twice a week.

And I don't go to any fast-food places at all any more, because there's really nothing I can have. My only big treat, once a month – I go to McDonald's and get a low-fat fruit yogurt. It has carbs in it, but I have it anyway. See, they don't tell you about the carbs. So it says 'low-fat' but there might be sugar in it. The fruit might have been frozen in sugar. They make you believe you're having something healthy, but you're not. You have to read every single ingredient before you buy anything. Like when I go to the supermarket, I buy the sugar-free lollies. When I want something sweet, I'll eat them. And if I have a bad night where I really crave something, I might eat three or four of them. But it gets me over that hump. I make sugar-free jelly. I buy diet drinks. I have one cup of coffee a day, in the morning.

Now I even try to eat breakfast. I'll have an egg and maybe two slices of bacon. Or I'll take cold meat and just roll it up with some low-fat cheese and a sliced tomato. I'm still not a big breakfast person. But I find that it gets the fire burning.

No baked goods. At work, if they bring in tuna on French bread, I might eat a little of the bread with the tuna. But the times I do that are very few and far between. I can't allow myself. Even now, I'm in a little bit of a stall. I've been yo-yo'ing with the same 10 pounds for the last three months. I was back home in Pennsylvania for three weeks, and I went to a wedding, a birthday party, and Thanksgiving – and I didn't gain anything. At my nephew's wedding I had the salmon, I ate the salad, and that was it. I didn't have any wedding cake.

On Thanksgiving my brother-in-law made me aubergine and I had salad. I didn't have the turkey and stuffing and potatoes and all that. My family's very supportive when I go home. And it felt good when I went back because I hadn't seen them for a while – at one point I lost 4 stone between visits, and the next time I saw them I had lost 2 more. By the time of my latest visit back home I had dropped about 9 stone. I was going to meet an old friend from high school for dinner, and he walked right past me. Then he turned around and said, 'Judy? You look no different than 25, 30 years ago.' I gave him the biggest kiss. I'm still heavy, don't get me wrong, but on this diet I went from a size 34 to a size 20. This is the only diet that has ever really worked for me.

how to eat in a restaurant

Because this diet is designed to be practical and user-friendly, it's easy to stick to the rules even if you dine out often.

This is not usually the case for weight-loss plans, which is why it was so important to us that the South Beach Diet work no matter who does the cooking. The dining out dilemma was especially painful for people on low-fat regimes. You either had to give the restaurant staff the third degree – What are the chicken breasts sautéed in? What exactly is in the vinaigrette? – or you had to bring your own food and hope no one objected. Even if they didn't, there was something sad about seeing healthy adults hovering over their Tupperware containers while their tablemates enjoyed fine dinners.

The overall trend in restaurant food over the past few decades has been towards healthy and fresh. Olive oil has become a staple. Every day it seems we read more about the benefits of certain fish. Menus include lots of grilled items and few that are fried. As a result, it's not hard to eat out when you're on the South Beach Diet.

Of course, you still have to watch what you're doing, but eating out is a good time to indulge in the things you love most, if only because doing so makes it a little easier to be moderate the rest of the time. There are a few strategies, many of which we've learned from patients, that can help you eat wisely even when you're on the town.

Here's a simple one: Eat something 15 minutes before you arrive at the restaurant. Just a little snack – a protein of some kind. A piece of low-fat cheese is good because you can carry it in your handbag or briefcase. It will begin the process of filling you up so that when it's time to order, you won't be feeling ravenous.

I recommend this also because it will help you get beyond the most treacherous part of any restaurant meal: the bread basket. Typically, you arrive, you're hungry, and there it is — fresh, perhaps warm and fragrant, and loaded with bad carbs. It won't really do much to satisfy your hunger, but it will jolt your bloodstream with glucose and set you up for reactive hypoglycemia and cravings for the rest of the evening.

Many people on the diet take the preemptive measure of telling the waiter to skip the bread basket altogether, which is a great idea as long as your fellow diners don't mind. If they do, you can always ask them to take their bread, *then* banish the basket.

Here's another good idea for the moment you arrive: Order soup, preferably a clear stock or consommé. The point of this, besides being filling, is that it extends your eating time. That's a good idea because there's a lag between when your belly begins to fill and when your brain notices it — maybe 20 minutes, the experts say. This fact explains why it's so easy to reach the point where you feel uncomfortably stuffed. Especially today, when speed is valued in both the preparation and the consumption of food, this is a danger. We eat so fast that we zoom right by the point of satiety and keep feeding ourselves until all of a sudden, we feel like we'll explode.

Starting a meal with stock begins the process of satisfying your hunger and initiates the signals to your brain that you are on the road to fullness. Anything that takes the edge off your hunger now is good, because it will keep you from eating more than you really need in a little while, when the food arrives.

If you peeped inside the bread basket and found a piece of the good, granary variety, you may decide to indulge yourself. If you do, dip it in olive oil, which will slow down the absorption of starches and contribute to your feeling of fullness. Believe it or not, bread with oil or even a little butter is better for your diet than bread alone, despite the fact that you're adding calories.

Here's another tip: Go to restaurants serving Mediterranean-style food. I don't just mean Italian — in fact, Italian restaurants can be dangerous because of how pasta and bread tend to dominate the meal. I'm thinking of Greek and Middle Eastern food. These are cuisines that employ lots of olive oil, which is always a plus. You can have hummus (paste made from chickpeas) on pitta bread, which is a *big* improvement over white bread and butter, and it's more flavoursome, too. You'll find good, whole grains such as tabouleh and couscous, which takes the place of potatoes or rice. And usually, these cuisines rely on spices and condiments rather than sweeteners to make the dishes taste good.

And if you *do* go Italian, try to structure the meal the way they do in Italy – in courses, with a modest serving of *al dente* pasta topped with a healthy tomato sauce, followed by a main course of meat or fish and fresh vegetables, including either leafy green ones like Batavian endive or spinach or crucifers like broccoli, plus a salad dressed in olive oil. In Italy, you don't sit down in front of a huge dish of pasta with a bottomless bread basket and call it dinner. That's why Italians can eat pasta twice a day and not suffer the obesity rates we see in the United States. In many restaurants you can request a half-portion of pasta as your appetizer. If you try this you'll see that it satisfies. It's important to eat enough good fats (the entrée and the olive oil) and good carbs (the vegetables and the salad) to counter the starches in the pasta.

We all tend to assume that restaurants serving Asian food are by definition healthy. The various Asian national diets tend to be heavy on fish and vegetables, light on heavy meats or sweets. But that's not always the case in Asian restaurants in Britain. One major difference is portion size – we are accustomed to a lot more food on our plates. And because everybody hates waste, we tend to finish what's there. Another significant difference is in the rice. Asians have always used the whole grain, meaning the fibre is there, too, and your digestive system has to work to get at the starch. In this country, and even increasingly in Asian cities, a more processed variety of white rice is used. That change substantially increases the glycemic load of a meal.

Something else you may not realize: MSG (monosodium glutamate), the flavouring agent, is made from beets, which are a healthy vegetable but have a very high glycemic index. They're loaded with sugar, in other words, though it is disguised fairly well in your average Chinese take-away dinner.

Stay away from rice or potatoes in *any* restaurant. Order a double serving of the vegetables instead. And never order anything that's fried. Roasted, grilled, braised, baked, steamed, even sautéed – all right. If there's a sauce, ask for it on the side – that doesn't mean you won't have any, but I guarantee that you'll be satisfied using half of what they would have ladled on.

As for drinks, start with water as soon as you're seated, but feel free to have a glass or two of red wine (which is actually good for your health and not terribly fattening) instead of white wine, spirits or, worst of all, beer.

For dessert, don't be too hard on yourself. If you eat out four times a week you need to say no most of the time, but if it feels like a special event, make the most of it. If fresh fruit would do the trick, have that. If fruit with ice-cream is what you need, that's fine, too. You can ask for them in separate dishes and make your own dessert, using three teaspoons of ice-cream topped by the fresh fruit. If only the most decadent chocolate cake will suffice, go ahead and order it – along with enough forks for everyone at the table. Have three bites only and eat them as slowly as possible. Then send the rest away with the first passing waiter. Try this experiment at home: Have three bites of any dessert, then stop and put the rest aside for a few minutes. You'll see that it was as satisfying as if you had eaten the whole thing. And you'll still respect yourself in the morning.

Of course, all this presupposes that you're eating in a normal, sit-down restaurant. But the fact is that most American dining out these days is done in fast-food places. It's hard to think of any strategy that might actually help there. Everything seems to conspire to deliver the worst meal possible, at least from our perspective.

Start by eliminating all the main attractions. No burgers (too many saturated fats in the meat and the cooking oil, too many carbs in the bun). No fish, either, since the coating and the cooking method make it even more fattening than the burger. No chips (the worst part of the meal from the glycemic index point of view, both the potatoes and the ketchup). No fizzy drink, which leads to pure sugar rush. Look at how fast-food restaurants emphasize their worse fare – even the offer to 'supersize' is simply a way to sell you excessive amounts of the cheapest part of the meal, the drink and the chips. The emphasis in fast food is on big, sweet, fat, and *fast* – everything that has made obesity such a problem in America today.

If you can visit a fast-food restaurant and limit yourself to salad (with oil and vinegar instead of any other dressing) and plain grilled chicken breast (in the places that serve it), accompanied by water or coffee, you can do all right. Chicken nuggets or fried chicken are bad news – like the fish, they consist of a lot of deep-fried bread over a little meat, which has been cooked in a trans fatty substance. Otherwise, you can't really eat at these places and follow any sort of healthful diet. That's no surprise, is it?'

MY SOUTH BEACH DIET

JUDITH W.:

I WENT DOWN THREE DRESS SIZES, AND MY CHOLESTEROL IS DOWN, TOO.

I 've had high blood pressure and angina for many years, and heart trouble runs in my family. I had a triple bypass in 1990, and I was the baby in the cardiac ward. My mother had already had one, and my sister had one, too. A few years ago I needed a new cardiologist and I went to Dr Agatston. The first thing he told me was that I had to lose weight, and since I weighed 12 stone at that time I knew he was right. He didn't tell me anything I didn't know. But he gave me the inspiration and he suggested this diet.

I cut out all of the carbs that I was supposed to cut out, and the sugar, too. They told me not to buy no-fat, because that just meant the foods were higher in sugars. But I did buy 2 percent milk and low-fat cheeses. Before I went on the diet, I never ate breakfast. But I would snack in the evening. I never snacked on sweets; it was always fruit or pretzels. I always ate baked potatoes, but never with butter, because I thought potatoes were all right. I'd have chips whenever I wanted. Of course I had a roll with my hamburger. I was trying to eat sensibly, but I wasn't really killing myself at it. And slowly but surely, I gained a lot of weight. I was in a panic when I started the diet, because I had never looked that big in my life. Never.

Once I got through the strict phase I began adding back some carbs. But not many. I don't trust carbs. I'll eat wholemeal pasta, but just a small amount. Brown rice, too. That's about it. Cheerios. No potatoes at all — only sweet potatoes. I bake them. I won't eat a whole potato, though — half. Sugar-free jams or jellies, if necessary, but I don't have a sweet tooth, so I'm lucky. When I added the carbs back, I still kept losing weight. I will now, occasionally, have a sandwich made with stone-ground wholemeal bread — thin-sliced, if I can get it.

I lost 2 stone over the course of maybe six months, and three years later I've kept it all off. I went down three dress sizes, and my cholesterol is down, too. My husband said it's the most expensive diet I ever went on, because I had to throw out all my clothes and start over. I'm an attorney, so I have a very expensive business wardrobe. And we go to a lot of evening functions, too. I love it – I finally have a great excuse for a whole new wardrobe.

back to cardiology

As I've noted, I came to study diet and weight loss only via my speciality of preventive cardiology. I fully agree with a quote from the famous Framingham Heart Study group: 'A heart attack or stroke should indicate a failure of medical therapy rather than the beginning of medical intervention.' I am convinced that preventing most heart attacks and strokes is not a pipe-dream but something that is feasible today. Even people who come to me with family histories of premature heart disease can, in most cases, overcome the genetic predisposition. The important thing is to begin prevention early. The earlier it is started, the easier it is to prevent future catastrophe. In too many cases, the first manifestation of heart attack or stroke is also the last.

Diet is, of course, a crucial component of our prevention strategy. For many patients, particularly those with diabetes or prediabetes, it is our primary focus. Exercise is important, but proper diet is absolutely the most essential element.

If you neglect that, you may someday have to take your chances with the so-called miracles of modern cardiology – angioplasty, coronary artery bypass, transplant, perhaps even the totally artificial heart. Such measures may restore sufficient cardiac function to keep you alive. These are the extreme, invasive, last-ditch efforts required once the patient and his or her doctors have proven unable to keep the cardiovascular system working as nature intended. In some cases there's a disease or dysfunction that caused the ailment. But overwhelmingly, most problems cardiologists treat can be *prevented*.

Exercise

As with diet, the goal here should be to find an exercise plan that will seem less like an intervention and more like part of your existing lifestyle – something you can incorporate easily into your routine. You can seek the greatest cardiac workout ever, one that will put you in marathoner shape. But if it requires you to remake your life it will probably be a flop. You'll never maintain it over the long haul, and the discouragement alone will leave you worse off than before you started.

Besides, you don't really *need* a Marine Corps-level exercise programme to have a healthy heart. What you need is a daily dose of activity that will achieve the desired effect as efficiently as possible. Anything beyond that is optional. Too many people approach this as an all-or-nothing proposition – they start out with a high-intensity programme, keep it up for a short spell, tire of it, and go back to doing nothing at all. Better to find a 30-minute workout you'll do daily. You won't burn a lot of calories each session, but the cumulative effect will be beneficial in every way. At the very least you'll offset the pound or two that most middle-aged people put on per year without even noticing. Clearly, people who exercise often and with gusto are better off than those who don't. It's not just a matter of cardiac health, either: Moving your body and pushing its limits puts you in a healthy frame of mind, I believe, in addition to the many other benefits.

The first thing you need is some kind of aerobic workout. You don't have to spend an hour on the treadmill, stair machine, elliptical trainer, or running track, however. Here's what I recommend: A brisk 20-minute walk every day. Don't run unless you really want to. Live by this easy-to-remember rule: As soon as you begin to perspire, you can call it quits. You get the majority of benefit from exercise during the first 20 minutes or so. If you want to stop at that point, it's all right. You've achieved your purpose. But you have to do it for 20 minutes, vigorously and religiously, every day. If you like swimming and it's possible to do it year round, be my guest. Again, you don't need to train like an Olympic hopeful. Twenty minutes.

In addition to that, I recommend some stretching, mainly because it ensures that you won't hurt yourself doing whatever other exercise you choose. But stretching is also good for circulation and lung function, which improves everything else. And it keeps your blood vessels young and healthy.

Finally, you need to do some weight training. It will improve your muscle–fat ratio, which will in turn raise your metabolism, causing your body to burn fuel faster even when you're asleep. You don't have to become a bodybuilder, but increasing lean body mass – meaning anything other than fat – is important. For women especially, weight training is good for how it builds bone density, which will forestall the effects of osteoporosis as you age.

In addition to all that, exercise lowers your blood pressure and bad cholesterol. Exercise regularly and eat properly, and you're doing just about all you can to ensure a healthy cardiac future. You're already doing far more for yourself than medical science can do for you.

Before a sustained workout (longer than 90 minutes), it may help to eat some low-glycemic carb, such as low-fat yogurt, porridge, or pumpernickel bread. Eat it at least two hours before exercising so you'll have a good supply of carbohydrates to give you an energy boost. After exercise you need to replenish glycogen fuel stores. You can even allow yourself white bread or potatoes at this time.

Medications and supplements

Earlier in the book, I described my journey as a cardiologist firmly committed to the 'prevention first' approach, especially as it pertains to diet. But nutrition and exercise alone can't always ensure cardiac health. In the late 1980s a new class of amazing cholesterol-lowering drugs known as the statins – medications such as Lescol, Zocor, and Lipitor – became available. With these, we were able to cut cholesterol quite easily and dramatically – 20 to 30 percent initially, and now, up to 50 percent. By taking these drugs, we thought, patients could have their cake and eat it, too – literally. They could diet or not and still enjoy low cholesterol. Of course, statins did nothing for the waistline. Still, the prevailing wisdom was to forget about diet and take the drugs. Statins were (and still are) expensive, and there is no research into the long-term effects of taking them. However, studies showed that the incidence of heart attacks could be diminished by approximately 30 percent with this class of medication.

I won't burden you with the scientific explanation behind statins. These compounds work by blocking the production of cholesterol in the liver. There has been some controversy associated with them, mainly over the possibility that they cause liver problems. One statin drug, Benecor, was withdrawn from the market after some patients taking it died of liver failure. There is no known problem with the statin drugs now on the market, however, despite the occasional scare that arises in the papers or on TV news shows. The benefits of statins far outweigh the potential hazards. Among physicians, there has never been any serious doubt about the wisdom of taking them. Consider this: Most cardiologists I know over the age of 40 are taking a statin drug, even doctors with no sign or history of heart trouble. The medication isn't cheap but the results are worth it.

Supplements, too, have become a big part of cardiac care in recent years.

Most people know to take an aspirin every day to thin the blood slightly and help prevent heart attack and strokes. It's worth emphasizing here what a blessing aspirin really is when it comes to cardiac prevention – it's so common and inexpensive that some people forget it's an important part of any heart-healthy regime.

For years we've been hearing how the classic antioxidant vitamins (A, C, and E) would help prevent heart attack, stroke, and cancer. Recently, though, multiple studies have failed to support these hopes with science. The good news is that vitamins and supplements don't do any harm (except to your wallet). The bad news is that they also appear to do no good. There's some evidence that the natural form of vitamin E, called d alpha tocopherol, is effective in preventing heart attacks and strokes. But further study is needed. My advice is to boost your body's supply of antioxidants by exercising and eating fruits and vegetables, which are rich in nutrients. I hedge my bet by suggesting a single daily multivitamin.

The news about taking fish-oil supplements, in capsule form, continues to be good, however. Just as we advise people to eat plenty of fish high in beneficial omega-3 oils, such as salmon and tuna, we suggest these capsules. They lower triglycerides and make the blood cells less sticky. They've also been found to prevent sudden death due to cardiac arrhythmia – the sudden, potentially fatal stoppage of the normal heartbeat. (For more on the marvels of fish oil, read Dr Andrew L. Stoll's excellent book, The Omega-3 Connection.)

I, personally, take one aspirin, two fish oil capsules, a statin drug, and an angiotensin-converting enzyme inhibitor, commonly known as an ACE inhibitor, which prevents inflammation, daily.

Recently, a study turned up another potentially important addition to the list of supplements. Some men undergo a kind of menopause equivalent associated with the normal drop in their testosterone levels starting in their fifties. We've always known that this hormone fuels sex drive. Now we find that it may also have something to do with cardiac function. Studies now indicate that men who have heart attacks often are found to have lower-than-normal testosterone levels. Diabetic men, too, tend to have low testosterone. Injections of this hormone in men who make no change in diet still results in lessened central obesity – it now seems as though the drop in testosterone may be another reason men gain weight as they age.

We never knew any of this before because we measured testosterone only in men with sexual dysfunction. Now we see the impact this hormone has on the entire obesity–cardiac health connection. I test for it in all my male patients and prescribe a testosterone gel (which is rubbed on the skin) for those whose levels are low.

Advanced blood testing

Lowering total cholesterol is an important goal in preventive care, but it's not nearly enough. In fact, most people who suffer heart attacks have average cholesterol levels. The fact is that one person can have a low cholesterol number and be at grave risk of a heart attack, while someone else with a higher figure will be fine. The familiar total cholesterol figure *alone* doesn't tell the entire story.

By now, most people will realize there are two basic types of cholesterol – the so-called good kind (high-density lipoproteins, or HDLs) and the bad (low-density, or LDLs). The ratio of good to bad is an important factor, one which is today commonly measured by diagnostic blood work.

But there are also other factors that must be considered, and for this reason advanced lipid testing has now become a requirement in any serious cardiac care.

The most sophisticated blood labs are now capable of measuring five different subgroups of HDL and seven of LDL. One thing they evaluate is the *size* of the cholesterol particles. In essence, large particles are good and small ones are bad. Large HDLs have proved to be more efficient at their job of clearing away bad fats than small HDLs are. Even more important, though, is the difference between large and small LDL particles.

The small ones squeeze more easily under the lining of blood vessels, where they form the plaque that narrows arteries. Larger LDL particles can't slide beneath the linings so well, and as a result their potential for harm is smaller.

Advanced blood lipid testing has been pioneered by the Lawrence Berkeley National Laboratory of the University of California at Berkeley and its commercial arm, the Berkeley HeartLab. Dr Robert Superko, medical director of the lab, has done an outstanding job of educating doctors in the use of advanced blood testing for treating patients. When the cholesterol sub-classes are taken along with other advanced tests, including Lp(a), homocysteine, and others, we can explain over 90 percent of the heart disease we see. We can also test for high sensitivity to C-reactive protein – CRP – a marker for inflammation of the blood vessel lining. Dr Paul Ridker, of Harvard, did the groundbreaking research proving that inflammation of the arteries can play a big role in arteriosclerosis and heart attacks. Measuring this inflammation can predict who is a candidate for a heart attack, even in patients with normal or low cholesterol. It's interesting to note that people with prediabetes or diabetes often have normal cholesterols but high CRPs.

EBT scanning

There's a final medical measure that must be taken to promote heart health, one with which I am extremely familiar: the use of electron beam tomography (EBT) as a non-invasive tool for examining the heart while it does its job. More than the electrocardiograph (ECG) or even the CT scan, this technology has the power to tell us the exact condition of the organ itself and the blood vessels that serve it. We can obtain critical information using this that no other diagnostic tests provide.

In June of 1988, I worked with my colleagues Warren Janowitz, David King, and Manuel Viamonte to come up with a method of identifying cardiac plaque simply, accurately, and painlessly, without having to invade the body. We used a then-revolutionary type of CT scan called electron beam tomography, or EBT.

This fast (5 minutes), painless (no needles or dye, no undressing) CT scanner was developed by a brilliant physicist, Douglas Boyd. The procedure takes pictures in a fraction of a second, freezing the image of the beating heart. With a conventional CT scanner the beating heart shows up as a blur. With General Electric's EBT, high resolution of the coronary arteries can be obtained, allowing us to see and measure calcium deposits, which are accurate indicators of the total amount of arteriosclerosis inside the vessel walls. Using these images we can identify who needs to be treated in advance of a heart attack or stroke. By treating the patient with diet, exercise, and medication, we can retest and monitor the effectiveness of the treatment.

Proper diet and exercise are still the most important things you can do to take care of your heart. Combine those with advanced lipid testing, aggressive lipid controls (statins and supplements), and the EBT, and the vast majority of heart attacks and even strokes can be averted.

MY SOUTH BEACH DIET

NANCY A.:

I DIDN'T GAIN ANYTHING DURING PREGNANCY.

I was working at Mount Sinai Hospital, in the child-care centre, where some of the children's parents work in the cardiovascular department. They invited us to be part of some research they were doing, and in exchange we'd get free diet consultations for three months. We had to pick a diet at random, and I ended up with the modified carbohydrate diet, which later became known as the South Beach Diet.

When I started I weighed 12 stone. For the previous five years, I had tried everything to lose weight. I tried appetite suppressant drugs three separate times. That's how I gained so much weight – I gained everything back double every time I stopped. I tried Slim-Fast, too. After a while I was getting really hungry from just drinking shakes, and so I went back to my regular eating habits. On my own, I decided to do salads only. That didn't work, either – I didn't have enough willpower. I would get even hungrier after eating a salad.

I'm Spanish, so we were raised on Spanish foods, which tend to have a lot of fat. I had to cut down on that stuff, fried foods especially. But every time I went a month or two eating healthy foods, I would crave my traditional dishes. Pork in the oven with rice, fried plantains, fried chicken. I couldn't stop myself from wanting it. I'm also a sweets person, so cheesecake here and there, a biscuit here and there. I work in a child-care centre, so we have tons of snacks for the children. After a big dinner, I would eat a bowl of ice-cream, or cereal, or cake.

The first two weeks on the South Beach Diet were the toughest – just low-fat meats and vegetables and water. Around the second week, I was going crazy. It was psychologically stressful. But I did it. Going to visit the nutritionist was helpful. Within those first weeks I think I cheated once, on cheesecake. A couple of times I was tempted to have rice, but I had stopped buying it, so there was none in the house. It kind of killed me, not having it around.

After the two strict weeks were up, it got a lot easier. I was able to have more variety. I went to the store and went crazy buying everything that was on the list. I was able to have fruit. And vegetables – I even started eating ones I'd never tried before. I was so eager to have more variety. Broccoli. Asparagus. Anything I saw.

After the three-month period, I had got down from around 12 to 10 stone. Actually, on the day I made the final visit to the nutritionist, I found out that I was pregnant. And I had been trying for five years. In fact, I had given up trying. And here I was, pregnant at last. I don't actually know what triggered that, but I think it's because I had been so overweight and not eating right. Something must have changed. And I had a perfect pregnancy.

I kept the weight off for two years. I didn't gain anything during the pregnancy. And only recently did I start to slide backwards. I've been neglecting myself a little, and some of the weight is back on. When you have a three-year-old and you're working at a day-care centre, you're surrounded by sweets. But I just got another copy of the diet from the nutritionist, and I'm going back again.

part two

Meal Plans and Recipes

phase 1 meal plan

This, as you know by now, is the strictest phase of the diet. It's meant to last for two weeks only – just long enough to resolve the insulin resistance that was brought about by eating too many bad (mostly processed) carbs. Phase I does not have to be low carb if you eat the right carbs. It is designed to allow ample portions of protein, good fats, and the lowest-glycemic index carbs needed for satisfaction and blood sugar control. These include the low-glycemic index vegetables, which also contribute fibre, important nutrients such as heart-healthy folic acid, and other vitamins and minerals. Many salads and vegetables are unlimited. You will also have your choice of proteins from a variety of sources.

By the time this phase ends, your unhealthy cravings, especially for sweets, baked goods, and starches, will also essentially have vanished. Even though this is the strict phase, you'll notice that each day includes six different occasions to eat – three meals, snacks in mid-morning and mid-afternoon, and dessert after dinner. So you should never feel hungry, and if you do, it's possible that you're being too stingy with your portions. The South Beach Diet doesn't require you to measure what you eat in ounces, calories, or anything else – the meals should be of normal size, enough to satisfy your hunger but no more than that.

Not all dinner recipes from the meal plans are included. Where there is no recipe to follow, chicken, fish or steak is the basis of the meal.

DAY ONE

Breakfast

- 150ml (6 fl oz) vegetable juice cocktail
- 2 Vegetable Quiche Cups To Go
- Decaffeinated coffee or decaffeinated tea with skimmed milk and sugar substitute

Mid-morning snack

- 1 chunk low-fat cheese

Lunch

- Sliced grilled chicken breast on lettuce
- 2 tablespoons Balsamic Vinaigrette or low-sugar prepared dressing
- Sugar-free jelly

Mid-afternoon snack

- Celery stuffed with 1 wedge Laughing Cow Light Cheese

Dinner

- Grilled Salmon with Rosemary
- Steamed asparagus
- Tossed salad (mixed leaves, cucumbers, green peppers, cherry tomatoes)
- Olive oil and vinegar to taste or 2 tablespoons low-sugar prepared dressing

Dessert

- Vanilla Ricotta Crème

DAY TWO

Breakfast

- 175ml (6 fl oz) tomato juice
- 1 egg
- 2 slices lean bacon
- Decaffeinated coffee or decaffeinated tea with skimmed milk and sugar substitute

Mid-morning snack

- 1–2 Turkey Roll-Ups
- 2 tablespoons Coriander Mayonnaise (optional)

Lunch

- South Beach Chopped Salad with Tuna
- Sugar-free jelly

Mid-afternoon snack

- Celery stuffed with 1 wedge Laughing Cow Light Cheese

Dinner

- Baked chicken breast
- Roasted Aubergine and Peppers
- Tossed salad (mixed leaves, cucumbers, green peppers, cherry tomatoes)
- 2 tablespoons Balsamic Vinaigrette or low-sugar prepared dressing

Dessert

- Mocha Ricotta Crème

DAY THREE

Breakfast

- 150ml (6 fl oz) vegetable juice cocktail
- Easy Asparagus and Mushroom Omelette
- Decaffeinated coffee or decaffeinated tea with skimmed milk and sugar substitute

Mid-morning snack

- 1 chunk low-fat cheese

Lunch

- Dilled Prawn Salad with Herb-Dill Dressing
- Sugar-free jelly

Mid-afternoon snack

- 1–2 Ham Roll-ups
- 2 tablespoons Coriander Mayonnaise (optional)

Dinner

- Grilled sirloin steak
- Steamed broccoli
- Grilled Tomatoes
- Mashed Cauliflower

Dessert

- Almond Ricotta Crème

DAY FOUR

Breakfast

- 175ml (6 fl oz) tomato juice
- Eggs Florentine (1 poached egg served on 100g (4 oz) spinach sautéed in olive oil)
- 2 slices lean bacon
- Decaffeinated coffee or decaffeinated tea with skimmed milk and sugar substitute

Mid-morning snack

- Celery stuffed with 1 wedge Laughing Cow Light Cheese

Lunch

- Chef's salad (at least 25g (1 oz) each ham, turkey, and low-fat cheese on mixed leaves)
- Olive oil and vinegar to taste or 2 tablespoons low-sugar prepared dressing

Mid-afternoon snack

- Up to 10 cherry tomatoes stuffed with 100g (4 oz) low-fat cottage cheese

Dinner

- White Fish in Spring Onion and Ginger Sauce
- Steamed mange-tout
- Shredded cabbage sautéed in olive oil

Dessert

- Mocha Ricotta Crème

DAY FIVE

Breakfast

- 150ml (6 fl oz) vegetable juice cocktail
- Western Egg White Omelette
- Decaffeinated coffee or decaffeinated tea with skimmed milk and sugar substitute

Mid-morning snack

- 1–2 Turkey Roll-ups
- 2 tablespoons Coriander Mayonnaise (optional)

Lunch

- Gazpacho
- Grilled sirloin hamburger steak (no bun)
- Tossed salad (mixed leaves, cucumber, green peppers, cherry tomatoes)
- Olive oil and vinegar to taste or 2 tablespoons low-sugar prepared dressing

Mid-afternoon snack

- Cucumber rounds with salmon spread

Dinner

- Balsamic Chicken
- Stewed Tomatoes and Onions
- Steamed spinach
- Tossed salad (mixed leaves, cucumber, green peppers, cherry tomatoes)
- Olive oil and vinegar to taste or 2 tablespoons low-sugar prepared dressing

Dessert

- Almond Ricotta Crème

DAY SIX

Breakfast

- 150ml (6 fl oz) tomato juice
- Scrambled eggs with fresh herbs and mushrooms
- 2 slices lean bacon
- Decaffeinated coffee or decaffeinated tea with skimmed milk and sugar substitute

Mid-morning snack

- 1 chunk low-fat cheese

Lunch

- Chicken Caesar salad (no croutons)
- 2 tablespoons prepared Caesar dressing

Mid-afternoon snack

- 100g (4 oz) low-fat cottage cheese with 50g (2 oz) chopped tomatoes and cucumber

Dinner

- Mahi.mahi or swordfish
- Oven-roasted Vegetables
- Rocket salad
- 2 tablespoons Balsamic Vinaigrette or low-sugar prepared dressing

Dessert

- Lemon Zest Ricotta Crème

DAY SEVEN

Breakfast

- 150ml (6 fl oz) vegetable juice cocktail
- Smoked Salmon Frittata
- Decaffeinated coffee or decaffeinated tea with skimmed milk and sugar substitute

Mid-morning snack

- Celery stuffed with 1 wedge Laughing Cow Light Cheese

Lunch

- Crab Cobb Salad
- Sugar-free jelly

Mid-afternoon snack

- 2 slices low-fat (light) mozzarella cheese with 2 slices fresh tomato sprinkled with balsamic vinegar, olive oil, and freshly ground black pepper

Dinner

- Marinated Grilled Steak
- Spinach-stuffed Mushrooms
- Mashed Cauliflower
- Tossed salad (mixed leaves, cucumber, green peppers, cherry tomatoes)
- Olive oil and vinegar to taste or 2 tablespoons low-sugar prepared dressing

Dessert

- Lime Zest Ricotta Crème

DAY EIGHT

Breakfast

- Light Spinach Frittata with Tomato Salsa
- Decaffeinated coffee or decaffeinated tea with skimmed milk and sugar substitute

Mid-morning snack

- 1 chunk low-fat cheese

Lunch

- Sliced steak (leftover Grilled Steak) on mixed leaves
- 2 tablespoons Balsamic Vinaigrette or 2 tablespoons low-sugar dressing
- Sugar-free jelly

Mid-afternoon snack

- Hummus with raw vegetables (you may use ready-made hummus)

Dinner

- Savoury Chicken Sauté
- Mashed Cauliflower
- Fresh steamed green beans
- Round lettuce and pecan salad
- Olive oil and vinegar to taste

Dessert

- Vanilla Ricotta Crème

DAY NINE

Breakfast

- 150ml (6 fl oz) vegetable juice cocktail
- 2 Vegetable Quiche Cups To Go
- Decaffeinated coffee or decaffeinated tea with skimmed milk and sugar substitute

Mid-morning snack

- 1–2 Turkey Rolls
- 2 tablespoons Coriander Mayonnaise (optional)

Lunch

- Greek Salad
- Sugar-free jelly

Mid-afternoon snack

- Celery stuffed with 1 wedge Laughing Cow Light Cheese

Dinner

- Fish Kebabs with Spaghetti Squash
- Sliced cucumber with olive oil

Dessert

- Lemon Zest Ricotta Crème

DAY TEN

Breakfast

- 175ml (6 fl oz) tomato juice
- Egg white omelette with chopped lean bacon and mushrooms
- Decaffeinated coffee or decaffeinated tea with skimmed milk and sugar substitute

Mid-morning snack

- 1 wedge Laughing Cow Light Cheese

Lunch

- Salad Niçoise

Mid-afternoon snack

- 75g (3 oz) low-fat cottage cheese

Dinner

- Cracked Pepper Steak
- Grilled Tomato with Pesto
- Steamed broccoli
- Mixed greens
- 2 tablespoons Balsamic Vinaigrette or low-sugar prepared dressing

Dessert

- Almond Ricotta Crème

DAY ELEVEN

Breakfast

- 175ml (6 fl oz) tomato juice
- Cheesy Frittata
- Decaffeinated coffee or decaffeinated tea with skimmed milk and sugar substitute

Mid-morning snack

- 1–2 Turkey Roll-ups
- 2 tablespoons Coriander Mayonnaise (optional)

Lunch

- Gazpacho
- Grilled sirloin hamburger steak (no bun)
- Tossed salad (mixed leaves, cucumber, green peppers, cherry tomatoes)
- Olive oil and vinegar to taste or 2 tablespoons low-sugar prepared dressing

Mid-afternoon snack

- Piece of fresh mozzarella cheese

Dinner

- Gingered Chicken Breast
- Steamed mange-tout
- Oriental Cabbage Salad

Dessert

- Almond Ricotta Crème

DAY TWELVE

Breakfast

- 150ml (6 fl oz) vegetable juice cocktail
- Broccoli and Ham Frittata
- Decaffeinated coffee or decaffeinated tea with skimmed milk and sugar substitute

Mid-morning snack

- 1 wedge Laughing Cow Light Cheese

Lunch

- Chicken-Pistachio Salad

Mid-afternoon snack

- Piece of fresh mozzarella cheese

Dinner

- Poached Salmon with Cucumber-Dill Sauce
- Green Bean Salad
- Grilled Tomatoes with Pesto
- Steamed asparagus

Dessert

- Lemon Zest Ricotta Crème

DAY THIRTEEN

Breakfast

- Baked eggs with lean, low-fat bacon strips
- Decaffeinated coffee or decaffeinated tea with skimmed milk and sugar substitute

Mid-morning snack

- Celery stuffed with 1 wedge Laughing Cow Light Cheese

Lunch

- Poached Salmon Spinach Salad (poached salmon left over from Day 12)
- Olive oil and vinegar to taste or 2 tablespoons low-sugar prepared dressing

Mid-afternoon snack

- Hummus with raw vegetables (you may use ready-made hummus)

Dinner

- Barbecued Steak with Tomato Relish

Dessert

- Mocha Ricotta Crème

DAY FOURTEEN

Breakfast

- Artichokes Benedict
- Mock Hollandaise Sauce
- Decaffeinated coffee or decaffeinated tea with skimmed milk and sugar substitute

Mid-morning snack

- 1–2 Turkey Roll-ups
- 2 tablespoons Coriander Mayonnaise (optional)

Lunch

- Red pepper stuffed with cottage cheese and chopped vegetables

Mid-afternoon snack

- Hummus with raw vegetables (you may use ready-made hummus)

Dinner

- Grilled chicken breast with plain grilled vegetables and fennel or endive

Dessert

- Sugar-free jelly with a tablespoon of low-fat topping or whipping cream with sugar substitute to taste

Foods to Enjoy

BEEF
Sirloin (including minced)
Tenderloin
Top round
Other lean cuts

POULTRY (SKINLESS)
Turkey and chicken breast
Poussin
Turkey bacon (2 slices per day)

SEAFOOD
All types of fish and shellfish

PORK
Boiled ham
Lean bacon
Tenderloin

VEAL
Leg cutlet
Top round
Veal chop

LUNCHMEAT
Nonfat or lower fat only

CHEESE (FAT-FREE OR LOWER FAT)
American
Cheddar
Feta
Mozzarella
Parmesan
Ricotta
Provolone

String
Dairy-free cream cheese substitute
1–2% or fat-free cottage cheese

NUTS
30 pistachios
20 small peanuts
15 pecan halves
1 teaspoon peanut butter

EGGS
The use of whole eggs is not limited unless otherwise directed by your doctor.
Use of egg whites as desired.

TOFU
Use soft, low-fat, or lite varieties

VEGETABLES
Alfalfa sprouts
Artichokes
Asparagus
Aubergines
Beans (black, butter, chickpeas, green, Italian, kidney, lentils, lima, pigeon, soy, split peas and wax)
Broccoli
Cabbage
Cauliflower
Celery
Collard greens
Courgettes
Cucumbers
Lettuce (all varieties)
Mushrooms (all varieties)

Snow peas
Spinach
Turnips
Water chestnuts

FATS
Canola oil
Olive oil

SPICES AND SEASONINGS
All spices that contain no added sugar
Broth
Extracts (almond, vanilla, etc.)

Horseradish sauce
Low-fat butter substitute
Pepper – black, cayenne, red, white

SWEET TREATS
Limit to 75 calories per day
Baking cocoa powder
No-added-sugar chocolate powder
Sugar-free ice-lollies
Sugar-free gelatin
Sugar-free hard sweets
Sugarless chewing gum
Sugar substitute

Foods to Avoid

BEEF
Brisket
Liver
Other fatty cuts
Rib steaks

POULTRY
Chicken wings and legs
Duck
Goose
Processed poultry products

PORK
Honey-baked ham

VEAL
Veal breast

CHEESE
Brie
Edam
Nonreduced fat

VEGETABLES
Beets
Carrots
Corn
Potatoes
Tomato (limit to 1 whole or 10 cherry per meal)
Sweet potatoes
Yams

FRUIT
Avoid all fruits and fruit juices in Phase 1, including:
Apples
Apricots
Berries
Cantaloupe
Grapefruit
Peaches
Pears

STARCHES AND CARBS
Avoid all starchy food in Phase 1, including:
Bread, all types
Cereal
Oatmeal
Rice, all types
Pasta, all types
Pastry and baked goods, all types

DAIRY
Avoid all dairy in Phase 1, including:
Frozen yogurt
Ice-cream
Milk
Soya milk
Yogurt

MISCELLANEOUS
Alcohol of any kind, including beer and wine

phase 1 recipes

Because this is the strictest phase, the palette of ingredients is relatively small. You'll be eating eggs for breakfast and lots of vegetables, low-fat cheeses, meat and fish the rest of the time. There's no bread, potatoes, fruit or rice during the first 2 weeks, true. But any plan that permits dishes such as Marinated Rump Steak, Crab Cobb Salad, Hummus and Lemon Zest Ricotta Crème can hardly be termed tough. And any programme that requires you to eat 6 times a day – 3 meals plus snacks in mid-morning and mid-afternoon, plus a nighttime dessert – is clearly meant to keep discomfort to a minimum.

BREAKFASTS

CHEESY FRITTATA

Serves 2

Lite cooking spray
2 teaspoons healthy butter-substitute spread
50g (2 oz) sliced onion
50g (2 oz) sliced red pepper
50g (2 oz) sliced courgette
2 small plum tomatoes, diced
1 tablespoon chopped fresh basil
Pinch freshly ground black pepper
2 eggs
100g (4 oz) virtually fat-free cottage cheese
50ml (2 fl oz) fat-free evaporated milk
20g (1¾ oz) grated reduced-fat Cheddar cheese

Coat an ovenproof 30cm (10-inch) frying pan with cooking spray and place over medium-low heat until hot. In the frying pan, melt the spread. Add the onion, red pepper, and courgette and sauté over medium-low heat until the vegetables are lightly browned, 2–3 minutes. Add the tomatoes, basil, and black pepper to the frying pan and stir to combine. Cook until the flavours are blended, 2–3 minutes, and remove from the heat.

Preheat the grill. In a blender, combine the eggs, cottage cheese, and milk and process until smooth. Pour the egg mixture over the vegetables. Cover and cook on medium-low heat until the bottom is set and the top is still slightly wet. Transfer the pan to the grill and grill until the top is set, 2–3 minutes. Sprinkle with the cheese and grill until the cheese melts.

Nutrition at a Glance

Per serving: 231 calories, 21g protein, 16g carbohydrates, 10g fat, 3g saturated fat, 480g sodium, 15mg cholesterol, 2g fibre

EASY ASPARAGUS AND MUSHROOM OMELETTE

Serves 1

3 stalks fresh asparagus
2 eggs
2 tablespoons water
Lite cooking spray
50g (2 oz) sliced white mushrooms
50g (2 oz) grated reduced-fat mozzarella cheese

Bring 2cm (1 inch) water to a boil in a large frying pan. Add the asparagus and cook, uncovered, just until tender. Meanwhile, in a medium bowl, whisk together the eggs and water. The whites and the yolk should be blended completely together.

Coat a 25cm (10-inch) non-stick frying pan with cooking spray. Heat the frying pan over medium-high heat until just hot enough to sizzle when a drop of water is added. Pour in the egg mixture. It should set immediately. With a spatula, lift edges as mixture begins to set to allow uncooked portion to flow underneath. When top is set, fill one half of the omelette with asparagus, mushrooms, and cheese. With the spatula, fold the omelette in half over the filling. Slide onto a serving plate. Serve immediately.

Nutrition at a Glance

Per serving: 238 calories, 21g protein, 5g carbohydrates, 15g fat, 6g saturated fat, 260mg sodium, 440mg cholesterol, 1g fibre

WESTERN EGG WHITE OMELETTE

Serves 1

Lite cooking spray
1 tablespoon chopped green pepper
1 tablespoon chopped spring onion
1 tablespoon chopped red pepper
2 eggs
3 tablespoons grated reduced-fat cheese

Lightly coat a medium frying pan with cooking spray. Sauté the green pepper, spring onion, and red pepper until they are slightly tender. Pour the eggs over the vegetables. When partially set, spread the cheese over half of the egg and fold the omelette. Continue cooking until cooked through.

Nutrition at a Glance

Per serving: 169 calories, 20g protein, 4g carbohydrates, 8g fat, 3g saturated fat, 320mg sodium, 15mg cholesterol, 1g fibre

VEGETABLE QUICHE CUPS TO GO

Serves 6

300g (10 oz) frozen chopped spinach
3 eggs
100g (4 oz) grated reduced-fat cheese
50g (2 oz) finely chopped green peppers
50g (2 oz) finely chopped onions
3 drops Tabasco sauce (optional)

Microwave the spinach for 2½ minutes on high. Drain excess liquid.

Line 12 muffin tins with baking cases.

Combine the eggs, cheese, peppers, onions, spinach, and Tabasco sauce if using, in a bowl. Mix well. Divide evenly among the muffin cases. Bake at 180°C/350°F/Gas 4 for 20 minutes until a knife inserted in the centre comes out clean.

Quiche cups can be frozen and reheated in the microwave. Any combination of appropriate vegetables and reduced-fat cheeses may be used.

Nutrition at a Glance

Per serving: 77 calories, 9g protein, 3g carbohydrates, 3g fat, 2g saturated fat, 160mg sodium, 10mg cholesterol, 2g fibre

ARTICHOKES BENEDICT

Serves 2

2 medium globe artichokes
2 slices lean bacon
2 eggs
4 tablespoons Mock Hollandaise Sauce (see opposite)

Wash the artichokes. Cut off the stems at the base and remove the small bottom leaves. Stand the artichokes upright in a deep saucepan with 5–7cm (2–3 inches) salted water. Cover and boil gently, 35–45 minutes. Turn the artichokes upside down to drain. Spread the leaves open like flower petals. With a spoon, carefully remove the centre petals and the fuzzy centre from the artichoke bottoms and discard. Keep the artichokes warm. Brown the bacon in a frying pan and poach the eggs in boiling salted water. Place a bacon slice into each artichoke top with a poached egg and Mock Hollandaise Sauce. Serve immediately.

Nutrition at a Glance

Per serving: 227 calories, 18g protein, 16g carbohydrates, 12g fat, 3g saturated fat, 540mg sodium, 225mg cholesterol, 8g fibre

MOCK HOLLANDAISE SAUCE

Serves 2

1 egg
1 tablespoon healthy butter-substitute spread
1 teaspoon fresh lemon juice
½ teaspoon Dijon mustard
Pinch paprika

In a 10 fl oz (½ pint) microwaveable liquid measure, combine the egg and the spread. Microwave on low (20%) for 1 minute, stirring once halfway through cooking, until the spread is softened.

Stir the lemon juice and mustard into the egg mixture and microwave on low for 3 minutes, stirring every 30 seconds, until thickened. Stir in the paprika. (If the mixture curdles, transfer to a blender and process on low speed for 30 seconds, until smooth.)

Nutrition at a Glance

Per serving: 54 calories, 4g protein, 2g carbohydrates, 4g fat, 0g saturated fat, 150mg sodium, 5mg cholesterol, 0g fibre

LUNCHES

GREEK SALAD

Serves 1

8 lettuce leaves, torn into bite-size pieces
1 cucumber, peeled, seeded, and sliced
1 tomato, chopped
50g (2 oz) sliced red onion
50g (2 oz) crumbled reduced-fat feta cheese
2 tablespoons extra-virgin olive oil
2 tablespoons fresh lemon juice
1 teaspoon dried oregano leaves
½ teaspoon salt

Combine the lettuce, cucumber, tomato, onion, and cheese in a large bowl.
Whisk together the oil, lemon juice, oregano, and salt in a small bowl.
Pour over the lettuce mixture and toss until coated.
This makes a nice accompaniment as a side salad for grilled chicken or fish.

Nutrition at a Glance

Per serving: 501 calories, 22g protein, 25g carbohydrates, 38g fat, 10g
saturated fat, 2300mg sodium (1134mg if salt omitted), 30mg cholesterol,
6g fibre

CHERRY SNAPPER CEVICHE

(Phase 1 Lunch or Dinner)

Serves 4

4 cherry snapper or trout fillets, coarsely chopped
3 fresh limes, juice of
½ teaspoon red chilli garlic paste (sambal oelek)
2 ripe plum tomatoes, coarsely chopped
½ yellow Spanish onion, coarsely chopped
2½ tablespoons fresh coriander, finely chopped
Sea salt
Black pepper

Soak the chopped fish in ¾ of the lime juice for 3 hours. Drain off the liquid and discard. Mix the fish with the red chilli garlic paste, tomatoes, onion, coriander, and the remaining lime juice. Season with salt and pepper to taste.

Nutrition at a Glance

Per serving: 225 calories, 36g protein, 15g carbohydrates, 2g fat, 1g saturated fat, 115mg sodium, 63mg cholesterol, 3g fibre

SOUTH BEACH CHOPPED SALAD WITH TUNA

Serves 1

Salad

  1 tin tuna chunks in brine (185g/6½ oz), drained and flaked
  75g (3 oz) chopped cucumber
  75g (3 oz) chopped tomato
  75g (3 oz) chopped avocado
  75g (3 oz) chopped celery
  75g (3 oz) chopped radishes
  1 handful chopped romaine lettuce

Dressing

  4 teaspoons extra-virgin olive oil
  2 tablespoons fresh lime juice
  2 cloves garlic, finely chopped
  ½ teaspoon crushed black pepper

To make the salad: Layer the tuna, cucumber, tomato, avocado, celery, radishes, and lettuce in a decorative glass bowl.

To make the dressing: Mix the olive oil, lime juice, garlic, and pepper. Drizzle over the salad.

Nutrition at a Glance

Per serving: 506 calories, 48g protein, 18g carbohydrates, 28g fat, 4g saturated fat, 640mg sodium, 50mg cholesterol, 6g fibre

CHICKEN-PISTACHIO SALAD

Serves 4

Salad

    50g (2 oz) shelled pistachio nuts, finely ground
    ½ + ¼ teaspoon salt
    ½ teaspoon + I pinch freshly ground black pepper
    4 boneless, skinless chicken breast halves
    2 tablespoons extra-virgin olive oil
    50g (2 oz) chopped sweet white onion
    I head romaine lettuce

Dressing

    I teaspoon grated sweet white onion
    I large ripe avocado, pitted and peeled
    3 tablespoons extra-virgin olive oil
    3 tablespoons fresh lime juice
    I tablespoon water

To make the salad: Preheat the oven to 190°C/375°F/Gas 5. Mix the nuts with ½ teaspoon salt and ½ teaspoon pepper in a pie dish. Press the chicken into the nuts. Heat I tablespoon of oil in a frying pan and cook the coated breasts, 2 minutes per side. Place the breasts in a baking dish, place in the oven, and bake for 15 minutes or until a thermometer inserted in the thickest portion registers 71°C (160°F) and the juices run clear.

Heat the remaining tablespoon of oil in a non-stick frying pan over high heat. Add the chopped onion, ¼ teaspoon salt, and a pinch of pepper. Cook until the onion is browned. Line 4 serving plates with lettuce.

To make the dressing: Purée the onion, avocado, oil, lime juice, and water in a blender.

Slice the chicken breasts and arrange I breast on top of the lettuce on each plate. Serve with the dressing.

Nutrition at a Glance

Per serving: 481 calories, 33g protein, 13g carbohydrates, 34g fat, 5g saturated fat, 520mg sodium, 70mg cholesterol, 5g fibre

DILLED PRAWN SALAD WITH HERB-DILL DRESSING

Serves 4

Prawns

225ml (8 fl oz) dry white wine
1 teaspoon mustard seeds
¼ teaspoon crushed red pepper
2 bay leaves
1 lemon, sliced
700g (1½ lb) large uncooked prawns (peeled and deveined)

Herb-Dill Dressing

3 tablespoons extra-virgin olive oil	1 teaspoon Dijon mustard
3 tablespoons red wine vinegar	½ medium onion, sliced
2 tablespoons water	1 large head romaine lettuce
2 tablespoons chopped fresh basil	4 ripe tomatoes, cut into wedges
2 tablespoons chopped fresh dill	6 fresh mushrooms, sliced
1 teaspoon finely chopped garlic	Fresh dill sprigs (optional)

To prepare the prawns: Combine the wine, mustard seeds, crushed pepper, bay leaves, and lemon in a large saucepan. Add water to fill pan two-thirds full. Bring to a boil over high heat, add prawns, and cook for 3–4 minutes or until prawns have turned pink and are no longer translucent in the centre. Drain and cool. Discard the bay leaves.

To make the herb-dill dressing: In a screw-top jar, mix the olive oil, red wine vinegar, water, basil, dill, garlic, mustard, and onion. Shake well.

Place the prawns in a large bowl and add the dressing. Toss well, cover, and refrigerate until well chilled. Serve the prawn mixture on romaine lettuce leaves and surround with tomato wedges and mushroom slices. Garnish with dill sprigs, if using.

Nutrition at a Glance

Per serving: 382 calories, 38g protein, 16g carbohydrates, 14g fat, 2g saturated fat, 310mg sodium, 260mg cholesterol, 4g fibre

CRAB COBB SALAD

Serves 2

6 handfuls romaine lettuce, torn into bite-size pieces
1 tin crabmeat (185g/6½ oz), drained
225g (8 oz) chopped ripe tomatoes or halved cherry tomatoes
50g (2 oz) crumbled blue cheese
2 tablespoons cholesterol-free bacon bits e.g. Bacos
50ml (2 fl oz) prepared low-sugar dressing or olive oil vinaigrette

Arrange the lettuce on a large serving dish. Arrange the crabmeat, tomatoes, blue cheese, and bacon bits in rows over the lettuce. Just before serving, drizzle some dressing evenly over the salad and toss well. Transfer to 2 chilled serving plates.

Nutrition at a Glance

Per serving: 267 calories, 27g protein, 12g carbohydrates, 13g fat, 4g saturated fat, 1012mg sodium, 95mg cholesterol, 4g fibre

SPICY TUNA

(Phase 1 Dinner)

Serves 4

50g (2 oz) white pepper
50g (2 oz) black pepper
50g (2 oz) fennel seeds
50g (2 oz) coriander seeds
50g (2 oz) ground cumin
2 tuna fillets (225g/8 oz each)
4 egg yolks
2½ tablespoons fresh coriander
2½ tablespoons fresh chives
2½ tablespoons parsley
4 deseeded green chillis
225ml (8 fl oz) rice vinegar
350ml (12 fl oz) olive oil
3 roasted red peppers
1 cucumber, finely sliced

In a preheated oven at 170°C/325°F/Gas 3, roast the white pepper, black pepper, fennel, and coriander for 15 minutes. Mix with the cumin and grind in a blender until finely ground.

Coat the tuna well with the roasted spices and pan sear until medium-rare. Set aside.

Make a chilli vinaigrette in a blender by mixing 2 of the egg yolks with the coriander, chives, parsley, and chillis and 100ml (4 fl oz) of rice vinegar. Add 150ml (6 fl oz) of oil slowly to emulsify.

Make a roasted pepper vinaigrette in a blender by mixing the remaining 2 egg yolks with the remaining 100ml (4 fl oz) of rice vinegar and the roasted red peppers, then emulsifying with the remaining oil.

Place the chilli vinaigrette and the roasted pepper vinaigrette on each half of a large dish. Slice the tuna and place on top of the vinaigrette. Garnish with the cucumber.

Nutrition at a Glance

Per serving: 626 calories, 37g protein, 57g carbohydrates, 26g fat, 4g unsaturated fat, 137mg sodium, 266mg cholesterol, 21g fibre

DINNERS

CHICKEN EN PAPILLOTE

Serves 4

4 boneless, skinless chicken breast halves (about 500g/1 lb)
Pinch salt
Pinch freshly ground black pepper
2 spring onions, chopped
1 medium carrot, sliced diagonally
1 small courgette, cut lengthwise in half, then crosswise into 1cm
   (½-inch) thick pieces
1 teaspoon dried tarragon
½ teaspoon grated orange zest

Heat oven to 200°C/400°F/Gas 6 (220°C/425°F/Gas 7 if foil is used). Cut four 60cm (2-foot) lengths of baking parchment or foil and fold each in half to make a 30cm (1-foot) square. Sprinkle the chicken breasts with salt and pepper. Place a breast slightly below the middle of each square of paper.

In a small bowl, combine the spring onions, carrot, courgette, tarragon, and orange zest. Spoon a quarter of the vegetable mixture over each chicken breast.

Fold the parchment or foil over the chicken, crimp edges together tightly, and bake for 20 minutes on a baking sheet. To serve, cut an X in the top of each packet with scissors and tear open.

Nutrition at a Glance

Per serving: 144 calories, 27g protein, 4g carbohydrates, 2g fat, 0g saturated fat, 86mg sodium, 65mg cholesterol, 1g fibre

BALSAMIC CHICKEN

Serves 6

6 boneless, skinless chicken breast halves
1 ½ teaspoons fresh rosemary leaves, finely chopped, or ½ teaspoon
   dried rosemary
2 cloves garlic, finely chopped
½ teaspoon freshly ground black pepper
½ teaspoon salt
2 tablespoons extra-virgin olive oil
Lite cooking spray
4–6 tablespoons white wine (optional)
75ml (3 fl oz) balsamic vinegar

Rinse the chicken and pat dry. Combine the rosemary, garlic, pepper, and salt in a small bowl; mix well. Place the chicken in a large bowl; drizzle with oil, and rub with the spice mixture. Cover and refrigerate overnight.

Preheat the oven to 230°C/450°F/Gas 8. Spray a heavy roasting pan or cast-iron frying pan with cooking spray. Place the chicken in the pan and bake for 10 minutes. Turn the chicken over, stirring in 3–4 tablespoons water or white wine (if using) if drippings begin to stick to the pan.

Bake for about 10 minutes or until a thermometer inserted in the thickest portion registers 71°C (160°F) and the juices run clear. If the pan is dry, stir in another 1–2 tablespoons of water or white wine to loosen drippings.

Drizzle the vinegar over the chicken in the pan. Transfer the chicken to plates. Stir the liquid in the pan; drizzle over the chicken.

Nutrition at a Glance

Per serving: 183 calories, 26g protein, 4g carbohydrates, 6g fat, 1g saturated fat, 270mg sodium, 65mg cholesterol, 0g fibre

DESSERTS

LEMON ZEST RICOTTA CRÈME

Serves 1

110g (4 oz) low-fat ricotta cheese
¼ teaspoon grated lemon zest
¼ teaspoon vanilla extract
1 sachet sugar substitute

Mix together the ricotta, lemon zest, vanilla extract, and sugar substitute in a dessert bowl. Serve chilled.

Nutrition at a Glance

Per serving: 178 calories, 14g protein, 7g carbohydrates, 10g fat, 6g saturated fat, 155mg sodium, 38mg cholesterol, 0g fibre

ALMOND RICOTTA CRÈME

Serves 1

110g (4 oz) low-fat ricotta cheese
¼ teaspoon almond extract
1 sachet sugar substitute
1 teaspoon slivered toasted almonds

Mix together the ricotta, almond extract, and sugar substitute in a dessert bowl. Serve chilled and sprinkled with toasted almonds.

Nutrition at a Glance

Per serving: 192 calories, 15g protein, 8g carbohydrates, 11g fat, 6g saturated fat, 155mg sodium, 38mg cholesterol, 0g fibre

VANILLA RICOTTA CRÈME

Serves 1

110g (4 oz) low-fat ricotta cheese
¼ teaspoon vanilla extract
1 sachet sugar substitute

Mix together the ricotta, vanilla extract, and sugar substitute in a dessert bowl. Serve chilled.

Nutrition at a Glance

Per serving: 178 calories, 14g protein, 7g carbohydrates, 10g fat, 6g saturated fat, 155mg sodium, 38mg cholesterol, 0g fibre

MOCHA RICOTTA CRÈME

Serves 1

110g (4 oz) low-fat ricotta cheese
½ teaspoon unsweetened cocoa powder
¼ teaspoon vanilla extract
1 sachet sugar substitute
Dash instant espresso powder
5 mini chocolate chips

Mix together the ricotta, cocoa powder, vanilla extract, and sugar substitute in a dessert bowl. Serve chilled with a dusting of espresso powder and sprinkle with the mini chocolate chips.

Nutrition at a Glance

Per serving: 261 calories, 15g protein, 17g carbohydrates, 14g fat, 9g saturated fat, 166mg sodium, 42mg cholesterol, 0g fibre

LIME ZEST RICOTTA CRÈME

Serves 1

110g (4 oz) low-fat ricotta cheese
¼ teaspoon grated lime zest
¼ teaspoon vanilla extract
1 sachet sugar substitute

Mix together the ricotta, lime zest, vanilla extract, and sugar substitute in a dessert bowl. Serve chilled.

Nutrition at a Glance

Per serving: 178 calories, 14g protein, 7g carbohydrates, 10g fat, 6g saturated fat, 155mg sodium, 38mg cholesterol, 0g fibre

phase 2 meal plan

We recommend that after two weeks of Phase 1, you switch to this, more liberal version of the diet. Here's where you begin to gradually reintroduce certain healthy carbs – fruit, granary bread, brown rice, wholemeal pasta, sweet potatoes – into your diet. The weight loss slows a little during Phase 2, which is why some dieters stay on Phase 1 longer than the 2-week period. If you're confident you can stick to that stricter plan for another week or two, feel free. But bear in mind that the relatively limited choices on Phase 1 make it a bad choice for a long-term diet – the danger is that you'll grow bored and be tempted to fall back into your old eating habits. You should stay on Phase 2 until you hit your target weight, at which point you move on to Phase 3. But there will be times during the course of your weight-loss regime that you will fall off the wagon – maybe you'll overindulge in sweets during a vacation, or around the holidays. Maybe there will be some stressful period that will lead you to put a few pounds back on. When that happens, we suggest that you switch back to Phase 1, just until you lose what you gained and get yourself back on track. That's how we designed the South Beach Diet – the three phases allow enough flexibility to accommodate real life.

Not all dinner recipes from the meal plans are included. Where there is no recipe to follow, chicken, fish or steak is the basis of the meal.

DAY ONE

Breakfast

- 150g (6 oz) fresh strawberries
- Oatmeal (100g (4 oz) old-fashioned oatmeal mixed with 225ml (8 fl oz) skimmed milk, cooked on low heat, and sprinkled with cinnamon and 1 tablespoon chopped walnuts)
- Decaffeinated coffee or decaffeinated tea with skimmed milk and sugar substitute

Mid-morning snack

- 1 hard-boiled egg

Lunch

- Mediterranean Chicken Salad

Mid-afternoon snack

- Fresh pear with 1 wedge Laughing Cow Light Cheese

Dinner

- Spinach-stuffed Salmon Fillet
- Vegetable Medley
- Tossed salad (mixed leaves, cucumber, green peppers, cherry tomatoes)
- Olive oil and vinegar to taste, or 2 tablespoons low-sugar prepared dressing

Dessert

- Chocolate-dipped Strawberries

DAY TWO

Breakfast

- Berry smoothie (225g (8 oz) fat-free fruit-flavoured yogurt, 75g (3 oz) berries, 75g (3 oz) crushed ice; blend until smooth)
- Decaffeinated coffee or decaffeinated tea with skimmed milk and sugar substitute

Mid-morning snack

- 1 hard-boiled egg

Lunch

- Lemon Couscous Chicken
- Tomatoes and cucumber slices

Mid-afternoon snack

- 110g (4 oz) fat-free yogurt

Dinner

- Meat Loaf
- Steamed asparagus
- Mushrooms sautéed in olive oil
- Sliced Spanish onion and tomato with drizzled olive oil

Dessert

- Slice of melon with 2 tablespoons ricotta cheese

DAY THREE

Breakfast

- 50g (2 oz) high-fibre cereal (such as Bran Flakes) with 150ml (6 fl oz) skimmed milk
- 110g (4 oz) fresh strawberries
- Decaffeinated coffee or decaffeinated tea with skimmed milk and sugar substitute

Mid-morning snack

- Small Granny Smith apple with 1 tablespoon peanut butter

Lunch

- Greek Salad

Mid-afternoon snack

- 110g (4 oz) fat-free yogurt

Dinner

- Herb-marinated Chicken
- Perfection Salad
- Steamed julienned courgette and yellow squash

Dessert

- Fresh pear with ricotta cheese and walnuts

DAY FOUR

Breakfast

- ½ fresh grapefruit
- I slice toasted wholemeal bread topped with 30g (I oz) sliced reduced-fat Cheddar cheese, grilled until cheese melts
- Decaffeinated coffee or decaffeinated tea with skimmed milk and sugar substitute

Mid-morning snack

- 110g (4 oz) fat-free yogurt

Lunch

- Chef's salad (at least 30g (I oz) each turkey, roast beef, and low-fat cheese on mixed leaves)
- 2 tablespoons Balsamic Vinaigrette or low-sugar prepared dressing

Mid-afternoon snack

- Small Granny Smith apple with I wedge Laughing Cow Light Cheese

Dinner

- Asian-style Chicken Packets with Vegetables
- Oriental Cabbage Salad

Dessert

- Almond Ricotta Crème

DAY FIVE

Breakfast

- Berry Smoothie (225g (8 oz) fat-free fruit-flavoured yogurt, 75g (3 oz) berries, 75g (3 oz) crushed ice; blend until smooth)
- Decaffeinated coffee or decaffeinated tea with skimmed milk and sugar substitute

Mid-morning snack

- 1 hard-boiled egg

Lunch

- Open-faced roast beef sandwich (75g (3 oz) lean roast beef, lettuce, tomato, onion, mustard, 1 slice granary bread)

Mid-afternoon snack

- 110g (4 oz) fat-free yogurt

Dinner

- Stir-fry Chicken and Vegetables
- Tossed salad (mixed leaves, cucumber, green peppers, cherry tomatoes)
- Olive oil and vinegar to taste or 2 tablespoons low-sugar prepared dressing

Dessert

- 110g (4 oz) fat-free, sugar-free dessert (e.g. Angel Delight) with 3–4 sliced strawberries

DAY SIX

Breakfast

- 150ml (6 fl oz) vegetable juice cocktail
- 1 poached egg
- 1 wholemeal muffin
- Decaffeinated coffee or decaffeinated tea with skimmed milk and sugar substitute

Mid-morning snack

- Small Granny Smith apple with 1 tablespoon peanut butter

Lunch

- 110g (4 oz) cottage cheese with ¼ cantaloupe melon, sliced
- 4 wholemeal biscuits
- Sugar-free jelly

Mid-afternoon snack

- Hummus with raw vegetables (you may use ready-made hummus)

Dinner

- Easy Chicken in Wine Sauce
- Italian-style Spaghetti Squash
- Rocket, spinach, and walnut salad
- Olive oil and balsamic vinegar to taste or 2 tablespoons prepared low-sugar dressing

Dessert

- Pistachio Bark

DAY SEVEN

Breakfast

- ¼ cantaloupe melon
- 1 slice toasted wholemeal bread topped with 30g (1 oz) sliced reduced-fat Cheddar cheese, grilled until cheese melts
- Decaffeinated coffee or decaffeinated tea with skimmed milk and sugar substitute

Mid-morning snack

- 110g (4 oz) fat-free yogurt

Lunch

- Tomato stuffed with tuna salad (90g (3 oz) tuna chunks in brine, 1 tablespoon chopped celery, 1 tablespoon mayonnaise), served on a bed of salad leaves

Mid-afternoon snack

- Aubergine and tahini with raw vegetables or wrapped in a lettuce leaf

Dinner

- Marinated Rump Steak
- Green and yellow French beans with red pepper sautéed in olive oil
- Mashed Cauliflower
- Tossed salad (mixed leaves, cucumber, green peppers, cherry tomatoes)
- Olive oil and vinegar to taste or 2 tablespoons low-sugar prepared dressing

Dessert

- Sliced cantaloupe melon with lime wedge

DAY EIGHT

Breakfast

- Sunrise Parfait
- Decaffeinated coffee or decaffeinated tea with skimmed milk and sugar substitute

Mid-morning snack

- 1 hard-boiled egg

Lunch

- Apple-Walnut Chicken Salad

Mid-afternoon snack

- 110g (4 oz) fat-free yogurt

Dinner

- Grilled Sole in Light Cream Sauce
- Grilled Tomato
- Butterhead lettuce salad
- Olive oil and balsamic vinegar to taste or 2 tablespoons prepared low-sugar dressing

Dessert

- Lemon Zest Ricotta Crème

DAY NINE

Breakfast

- Eggs Florentine (1 poached egg served on 110g (4 oz) spinach sautéed in olive oil)
- Decaffeinated coffee or decaffeinated tea with skimmed milk and sugar substitute

Mid-morning snack

- Small Granny Smith apple with 1 tablespoon peanut butter

Lunch

- Tomato-Basil Couscous Salad

Mid-afternoon snack

- 110g (4 oz) fat-free yogurt

Dinner

- Salsa Chicken
- Tossed salad (mixed leaves, cucumber, green peppers, cherry tomatoes)
- 2 tablespoons Balsamic Vinaigrette or 2 tablespoons prepared low-sugar dressing

Dessert

- Chocolate Cups

DAY TEN

Breakfast

- Oatmeal Pancake
- Decaffeinated coffee or decaffeinated tea with skimmed milk and sugar substitute

Mid-morning snack

- Small Granny Smith apple with 1 tablespoon peanut butter

Lunch

- Chicken and Raspberry Spinach Salad (cold chicken breast left over from Day 9)

Mid-afternoon snack

- 110g (4 oz) fat-free yogurt

Dinner

- Meat Loaf
- Italian-style Spaghetti Squash

Dessert

- Strawberries with sugar substitute of your choice or dollop of low-fat topping/cream

DAY ELEVEN

Breakfast

- 110g (4 oz) fresh strawberries
- 50g (2 oz) high-fibre cereal (such as Bran Flakes) with 150ml (6 fl oz) skimmed milk
- Decaffeinated coffee or decaffeinated tea with skimmed milk and sugar substitute

Mid-morning snack

- 1 hard-boiled egg

Lunch

- Turkey-tomato pitta (75g (3 oz) sliced turkey, 3 tomato slices, small handful shredded lettuce, 1 teaspoonful Dijon mustard in a wholemeal pitta)

Mid-afternoon snack

- 110g (4 oz) fat-free yogurt

Dinner

- Cod en Papillote
- Butterhead lettuce salad
- Olive oil and balsamic vinegar to taste or 2 tablespoons prepared low-sugar dressing

Dessert

- Baked apple

DAY TWELVE

Breakfast

- ½ grapefruit
- I egg, any style
- 2 slice multigrain bread
- Low-sugar jam or marmalade
- Decaffeinated coffee or decaffeinated tea with skimmed milk and sugar substitute

Mid-morning snack

- I chunk low-fat cheese

Lunch

- Tomato Soup
- Chopped sirloin beef patty with I slice tomato and I slice onion in ½ wholemeal pitta

Mid-afternoon snack

- Aubergine and tahini with raw vegetables or wrapped in a lettuce leaf

Dinner

- Grilled Chicken Salad with Tzatziki Sauce
- Grilled asparagus with drizzled olive oil
- Tossed salad (mixed leaves, cucumber, green peppers, cherry tomatoes)
- 2 tablespoons Balsamic Vinaigrette or 2 tablespoons prepared low-sugar dressing

Dessert

- Fresh pear with ricotta cheese and walnuts

DAY THIRTEEN

Breakfast

- 110g (4 oz) blueberries
- 1 scrambled egg with tomato salsa
- Oatmeal (60g (2 oz) old-fashioned oatmeal mixed with 225ml (8 fl oz) skimmed milk, cooked on low heat, and sprinkled with cinnamon and 1 tablespoon chopped walnuts)
- Decaffeinated coffee or decaffeinated tea with skimmed milk and sugar substitute

Mid-morning snack

- 110g (4 oz) fat-free yogurt

Lunch

- Tuna salad (80g (3 oz) tuna chunks in brine, 1 tablespoon chopped celery, 1 tablespoon mayonnaise, 3 slices tomato, 3 slices onion) in a wholemeal pitta

Mid-afternoon snack

- 1 chunk low-fat cheese

Dinner

- Pan-roasted Steak and Onions
- South Beach Salad
- Steamed broccoli

Dessert

- Chocolate-dipped Strawberries

DAY FOURTEEN

Breakfast

- 150ml (6 fl oz) vegetable juice cocktail
- Baked eggs in lean bacon cups
- 1 slice multigrain bread, toasted
- Decaffeinated coffee or decaffeinated tea with skimmed milk and sugar substitute

Mid-morning snack

- 110g (4 oz) fat-free yogurt

Lunch

- Portobello Pizza

Mid-afternoon snack

- Small Granny Smith apple with 1 wedge Laughing Cow Light Cheese

Dinner

- Grilled salmon
- Couscous
- White Asparagus Salad

Dessert

- Fresh Strawberries with Lime Zest Ricotta Crème

Foods to Reintroduce

FRUIT
Apples
Apricots (dried)
Apricots (fresh)
Blueberries
Cantaloupe
Cherries
Grapefruit
Grapes
Kiwi
Mangoes
Oranges
Peaches
Pears
Plums
Strawberries

DAIRY
Light fruit-flavoured yogurt
Light soya milk
Nonfat or 1% milk
Plain low-fat or fat-free yogurt

STARCHES
Use sparingly
All-Bran cereal
Bran Flakes cereal

Other high-fibre cereals
Oatmeal (not instant)
Sugar-free bran muffins (no raisins)
Brown rice
Wild rice
Wholewheat pasta
Wholewheat pittas
Stone-ground pittas
Multigrain bread
Oat and bran bread
Rye bread
Wholewheat bread
Small wholegrain bagels
Green peas
Small sweet potato
Popcorn

VEGETABLES AND LEGUMES
Black-eyed beans
Pinto beans
Barley

MISCELLANEOUS
Bittersweet chocolate (sparingly)
Semisweet chocolate (sparingly)
Fat-free sugar-free pudding
Red wine

Foods to Avoid or Eat Rarely

STARCHES AND BREADS
White rice
Baked white potatoes
Instant potatoes
Dinner rolls
Refined wheat bread
Refined wheat bagel
White bread
White flour pasta
Pretzels
Rice cakes
Cornflakes
Biscuits

VEGETABLES
Beetroot
Carrots
Corn
Potatoes

FRUIT
Bananas
Fruit juice
Juice-packed canned fruit
Pineapple
Raisins
Watermelon

MISCELLANEOUS
Honey/jam
Ice-cream

phase 2 recipes

Now that you've resolved your insulin resistance and lost a dozen or so pounds, you're ready to settle into a long-term weight loss programme. Phase 2 begins gradually reintroducing carbohydrates into your diet, starting with low-glycemic index ones such as oatmeal and couscous. The recipes herein still don't recommend even good high-glycemic carbohydrates, such as sweet potatoes, whole wheat pasta or whole grain bread or rice; the diet's flexibility allows you to begin adding these unprocessed carbs into your meals as you see fit. In this phase the desserts also become more liberal, allowing, for instance, Chocolate-dipped Strawberries.

BREAKFASTS

OATMEAL PANCAKE

Serves 1

60g (2 oz) old-fashioned oatmeal
60g (2 oz) low-fat cottage cheese (or tofu)
4 egg whites
1 teaspoon vanilla extract
¼ teaspoon cinnamon
¼ teaspoon nutmeg
Lite cooking spray

Mix the oatmeal, cottage cheese, egg whites, vanilla extract, cinnamon, and nutmeg in a blender until smooth. Spray a non-stick frying pan with cooking spray. Add the batter and cook over medium heat until both sides are lightly browned.

You can top the pancake with a low-sugar syrup of your choice.

Nutrition at a Glance

Per serving: 288 calories, 28g protein, 32g carbohydrates, 4g fat, 1g saturated fat, 451mg sodium, 5mg cholesterol, 5g fibre

SUNRISE PARFAIT

Serves 2

150g (6 oz) sliced strawberries
225g (8 oz) fat-free vanilla yogurt
50g (2 oz) Bran Flakes

Layer the strawberries, yogurt, and cereal in 2 stemmed dessert glasses.

Nutrition at a Glance

Per serving: 185 calories, 8g protein, 37g carbohydrates, 1g fat, 0g saturated fat, 102mg sodium, 3mg cholesterol, 6g fibre

LUNCHES

POACHED SALMON SPINACH SALAD

Serves 4

Poached salmon left over from Poached Salmon with Cucumber-Dill
  Sauce
2 tablespoons extra-virgin olive oil
225g (½ lb) cleaned fresh spinach
¼ teaspoon salt
⅛ teaspoon freshly ground black pepper
60g (2 oz) chopped onion
3 fresh tomatoes (about 550g/1¼ pounds), peeled, seeded and cut
  into 1cm (½ inch) pieces
1 tablespoon coarsely chopped flat-leaf parsley (optional)

Arrange the salmon on a plate. In a frying pan, heat 1 tablespoon of the oil
over medium heat. When hot, sauté the spinach for 1½ minutes. Mix in
the salt and pepper and divide the spinach among 4 plates. Heat the
remaining tablespoon of oil in the frying pan. Sauté the onion and
tomatoes over medium heat until the onion is tender, about 5–6 minutes.
Arrange the salmon on the spinach and top with the tomatoes and onion.
Garnish with parsley, if using.

Nutrition at a Glance

Per serving: 98 calories, 2g protein, 9g carbohydrates, 7g fat, 1g saturated
fat, 162mg sodium, 0mg cholesterol, 2g fibre

MEDITERRANEAN CHICKEN SALAD

Serves 6

Dressing

- 110ml (4 fl oz) low-sugar prepared Italian dressing
- 1 tablespoon hot Tabasco sauce
- ½ tablespoon dried mint leaves
- ¼ tablespoon mustard powder

Salad

- 450g (1 lb) boneless, skinless chicken breast
- 2 tablespoons extra-virgin olive oil
- 350g (12 oz) prepared bulgur wheat
- 150g (5 oz) chopped cucumbers
- 300g (10 oz) chopped tomatoes
- 115g (4 oz) finely chopped spring onions
- 30g (1 oz) chopped fresh parsley
- Romaine lettuce leaves

To make the dressing: Whisk together the dressing, Tabasco, mint, and mustard powder in a small bowl. Cover and chill until ready to use.

To make the salad: In a medium frying pan, cook the chicken in the oil over medium heat for 8–10 minutes or until the chicken is tender and no longer pink, turning often to brown evenly. Remove the chicken from the frying pan. Cut into thin, bite-size cubes. Allow the chicken to cool, then refrigerate until fully chilled. Combine the chicken with the bulgur, cucumbers, tomatoes, onions, and parsley in a bowl. Serve over the lettuce with the dressing.

Nutrition at a Glance

Per serving: 220 calories, 20g protein, 18g carbohydrates, 8g fat, 1g saturated fat, 279mg sodium, 45mg cholesterol, 4g fibre

TOMATO-BASIL COUSCOUS SALAD

Serves 6

150g (5 oz) cooked couscous
1 tomato, chopped
50g (2 oz) tinned chick peas, drained and rinsed
2 spring onions, chopped
1 teaspoon extra-virgin olive oil
1 tablespoon fresh lemon juice
1 tablespoon chopped fresh basil
Lettuce

Combine the couscous, tomato, chick peas, spring onions, oil, lemon juice, and basil in a bowl, toss, and serve on a bed of lettuce.

Nutrition at a Glance

Per serving: 43 calories, 2g protein, 7g carbohydrates, 1g fat, 0g saturated fat, 0mg sodium, 0mg cholesterol, 1g fibre

LEMON COUSCOUS CHICKEN

Serves 4

280ml (10 fl oz) water
1 tablespoon extra-virgin olive oil
350g (12 oz) broccoli florets
175g (6 oz) packet couscous (e.g. Waitrose Garlic and Coriander)
350g (12 oz) chopped cooked chicken
Juice of 1 lemon (about 3 tablespoons)
¼ teaspoon lemon zest

In a large frying pan, bring the water, oil, and broccoli to a boil. Stir in the couscous, chicken, lemon juice, and lemon zest. Remove from the heat. Cover and let stand for 5 minutes. Fluff lightly with a fork. Chill well and serve cold.

Nutrition at a Glance

Per serving: 311 calories, 24g protein, 39g carbohydrates, 7g fat, 1g saturated fat, 476mg sodium, 45mg cholesterol, 3g fibre

RUMI CHOPPED SALAD WITH LEMON VINAIGRETTE

Phase 2 Lunch or Dinner

Serves 1

Salad

  1 beetroot
  50ml (2 fl oz) sherry vinegar
  1 red pepper
  25g (1 oz) pecans
  25g (1 oz) kalamata olives
  6 basil leaves
  1 shallot

Vinaigrette

  50ml (2 fl oz) lemon juice
  Salt
  White pepper
  1 egg
  1 teaspoon Dijon mustard
  80ml (3 fl oz) olive oil
  80ml (3 fl oz) rapeseed oil
  1 head chicory, thinly sliced
  1 handful frisée leaves
  1 orange, peeled and sectioned

To make the salad: Roast the beetroot until tender and dice into small cubes. Place the excess beetroot juice in the sherry vinegar and cook to make a marinade. Strain beetroot marinade and cover the diced beetroot with it. Roast the pepper and dice. Roast the pecans and chop them, saving some whole for garnish. Cut the olives into slivers, slice the basil leaves into strips, and chop the shallot into small pieces.

To make the vinaigrette: Place the lemon juice, salt, pepper, egg, and mustard in a blender and mix. Add the olive oil and rapeseed oil slowly to create an emulsion.

Mix the chicory, frisée, orange, pepper, pecans, olives, basil, shallot, and vinaigrette. Place a mound of diced beetroot with the juice on a plate and place a mound of dressed salad on top of that. Garnish with a whole pecan.

Nutrition at a Glance

Per serving: 338 calories, 2g protein, 9g carbohydrates, 33g fat, 4g saturated fat, 120mg sodium, 35mg cholesterol, 3g fibre

PORTOBELLO PIZZA

Serves 2

1 teaspoon extra-virgin olive oil
1 clove garlic, roughly chopped
175g (6 oz) portobello mushroom caps, cleaned
Pinch salt
Pinch freshly ground black pepper
350g (12 oz) mozzarella cheese, sliced or grated
10 fresh basil leaves
2 fresh tomatoes, sliced, roasted, or grilled
Oregano leaves (optional)

Combine the oil and garlic in a small bowl and rub the mushroom caps with the mixture on all sides. Place the caps top side down to form a circle on an oiled baking sheet; season with the salt and pepper. Arrange the cheese, basil, and tomato slices alternately in a circle on top. Sprinkle with the oregano, if using. Bake at 230°C/450°F/Gas 8 until the cheese melts, about 3 minutes.

Nutrition at a Glance

Per serving: 549 calories, 36g protein, 14g carbohydrates, 40g fat, 23g saturated fat, 651mg sodium, 133mg cholesterol, 3g fibre

TOMATO SOUP

Serves 2

1 small onion, chopped
50g (2 oz) sliced mushrooms
80g (3 oz) diced ham
¼ teaspoon extra-virgin olive oil
1 clove garlic, finely chopped
⅛ teaspoon sweet paprika
Pinch allspice
425ml (15 fl oz) chicken stock
1 tin (400g/14 oz) chick peas
3 whole tomatoes, peeled

Mix the onion, mushrooms, ham, oil, garlic, paprika, and allspice in a large pan; cook for 1 minute. Add the chicken stock, chick peas, and tomatoes; cover and simmer for 15 minutes. Purée the soup in a blender.

Nutrition at a Glance

Per serving: 404 calories, 29g protein, 58g carbohydrates, 7g fat, 2g saturated fat, 1341mg sodium, 25mg cholesterol, 12g fibre

DINNERS

STIR-FRY CHICKEN AND VEGETABLES

Serves 4

3 tablespoons rapeseed oil

225g (½ lb) cooked chicken breast, cut diagonally into 3mm (⅛ inch) thick slices

300g (10 oz) mixed prepared vegetables including broccoli, green beans, red peppers, and mushrooms

2 tablespoons water

2 tablespoons soy sauce

300g (10 oz) fresh spinach

Heat a large, heavy frying pan or wok over high heat until water sizzles when dropped onto the metal. Add 1½ tablespoons of the oil and tilt the pan gently in all directions until the oil has coated the surface. When the oil is hot (not to the point of smoking), add the chicken breast slices and stir-fry for 2 minutes. Remove the chicken to a bowl. Add the remaining oil to the frying pan. When hot, add the vegetables and stir-fry for about 4 minutes, until the larger pieces are cooked through. Return the chicken to the frying pan, add the water and soy sauce, and stir-fry for an additional 2 minutes. Add the spinach. Cover the pan and steam over medium heat for 2 minutes. Using tongs, turn the spinach once, so that it heats evenly; cover and steam for an additional 2 minutes. Remove the chicken and vegetables with a slotted spoon. Spoon the liquid into small bowls and serve as a gravy or dip.

Nutrition at a Glance

Per serving: 232 calories, 23g protein, 7g carbohydrates, 13g fat, 2g saturated fat, 616mg sodium, 48mg cholesterol, 4g fibre

EASY CHICKEN IN WINE SAUCE

Serves 4

4 tablespoons extra-virgin olive oil
1 clove garlic, crushed
3 boneless, skinless chicken breast halves, cut into strips
⅛ teaspoon salt
¼ teaspoon coarsely ground black pepper
100ml (4 fl oz) dry white wine
3 medium tomatoes, sliced

In a medium frying pan, heat the oil and garlic over medium heat; sprinkle the chicken with the salt and pepper, then add to the frying pan and cook for 7–10 minutes. Add the white wine and cook for an additional 2 minutes.

Remove the chicken and place on a dish; place the tomatoes in the frying pan and sauté until tender. Place the tomatoes over the chicken and cover with the pan drippings.

Nutrition at a Glance

Per serving: 190 calories, 6g protein, 5g carbohydrates, 15g fat, 2g saturated fat, 117mg sodium, 12mg cholesterol, 1g fibre

DESSERTS

CHOCOLATE-DIPPED STRAWBERRIES

Serves 2

2 squares (25g/1 oz each) dark chocolate, chopped
½ tablespoon whipping cream
Dash almond extract
8 strawberries

Combine the chocolate and the whipping cream in a glass measuring cup or bowl. Microwave at medium power for 1 minute or until the chocolate melts, stirring after 30 seconds. Stir in the almond extract and let cool slightly.

Dip each strawberry into the melted chocolate, allowing the excess to drip off. Place on a greaseproof paper-lined baking sheet. Refrigerate or freeze for approximately 15 minutes until set.

Nutrition at a Glance

Per serving: 175 calories, 3g protein, 24g carbohydrates, 9g fat, 6g saturated fat, 1mg sodium, 5mg cholesterol, 4g fibre

STRAWBERRIES WITH LIGHT VANILLA YOGURT

Serves 1

110g (4 oz) fat-free vanilla yogurt
110g (4 oz) chopped strawberries

Spoon the yogurt into a dessert bowl, then add the strawberries. Serve immediately.

Nutrition at a Glance

Per serving: 85 calories, 4g protein, 16g carbohydrates, 0g fat, 0g saturated fat, 66mg sodium, 3mg cholesterol, 2g fibre

PISTACHIO BARK

Makes 450g (1 lb); serves about 18

12 squares dark chocolate
150g (5 oz) pistachio nuts, shelled and toasted

Microwave the chocolate in a microwaveable bowl on high for 2 minutes, stirring halfway through. Stir until completely melted. Stir the nuts into the chocolate. Spoon the chocolate and nut mixture onto a greaseproof paper-lined baking sheet. Refrigerate for 1 hour until firm. Break into bite-size pieces.

Nutrition at a Glance

Per serving (25g/1 oz): 150 calories, 3g protein, 16g carbohydrates, 10g fat, 4g saturated fat, 0mg sodium, 0mg cholesterol, 2g fibre

CHOCOLATE CUPS

Serves 8

Chocolate Cups
   8 fluted paper baking cups (to fit 8cm (3 in) muffin pan cups)
   450g (1 lb) semisweet chocolate pieces
   1 tablespoon low-fat margarine

Filling
   1 packet (85g/3½ oz) sugar-free vanilla-flavoured pudding mix (e.g.
     Angel Delight)
   285ml (½ pt) skimmed milk or as directed
   Cocoa powder

To make the Chocolate Cups, first place a paper baking cup in each of the
8 cups of the muffin pan; set aside.

In a double boiler over hot, not boiling, water (or in heavy saucepan
over a low heat), heat the chocolate pieces with the margarine until
melted and smooth, about 5 minutes, stirring occasionally.

Starting from the top rim of each paper cup, drizzle the chocolate
mixture, 1 heaped teaspoon at a time, down the side of the cup. About 3
of these teaspoonfuls will cover the entire inside of each cup. Refrigerate
until chocolate is firm, about 30 minutes.

Prepare the pudding using the milk. With a rubber spatula, fold in the
whipped topping. Spoon the cream filling into the chocolate cups; sprinkle
with cocoa powder.

Nutrition at a Glance

Per serving: 99 calories, 2g protein, 17g carbohydrates, 3g fat, 1g saturated
fat, 206mg sodium, 5mg cholesterol, 0g fibre

phase 3 meal plan

By now you should be at your ideal weight. If you've stuck with the diet, your blood chemistry should also be improved. This is the part of the plan that's meant to help you maintain the benefits you've earned by following Phases 1 and 2. This is how you'll eat for the rest of your life. Phase 3 is the most liberal stage of the diet – by now it is simply one important aspect of a healthy lifestyle rather than a weight-loss pro-gramme. At this point you should be knowledgeable enough about how the South Beach Diet works and how it interacts with your own body to enjoy all the flexibility of the plan. In other words, if you want it, and it doesn't undo all your sacrifices, you should go ahead and enjoy. There will always be times when you overindulge a little, even after years on the diet. Those are the times when you'll switch back to Phase 1 for a week or two. You'll get back to where you were, and then you'll return to Phase 3. Don't even think of it as backsliding – we designed the diet to allow normal human beings to eat the way they want. If for you, that means having a few too many desserts once in a while, great. Enjoy it.

Not all dinner recipes from the meal plans are included. Where there is no recipe to follow, chicken or poussin (baby chicken available from supermarkets), fish or steak is the basis of the meal.

DAY ONE

Breakfast

- ½ grapefruit
- 2 Vegetable Quiche Cups To Go
- Oatmeal (60g/2 oz old-fashioned oatmeal mixed with 225ml (8 fl oz) skimmed milk, cooked on low heat, and sprinkled with cinnamon and 1 tablespoon chopped walnuts)
- Decaffeinated coffee or decaffeinated tea with skimmed milk and sugar substitute

Lunch

- Roast Beef Wrap
- Fresh apple

Dinner

- Moroccan Grilled Chicken
- Steamed asparagus
- Couscous
- Mediterranean Salad
- Olive oil and vinegar to taste or 2 tablespoons low-sugar prepared dressing

Dessert

- Strawberries with Light Vanilla Yogurt

DAY TWO

Breakfast

- Fresh orange, sliced
- 1 egg
- 2 slices lean bacon
- 1 slice granary bread
- Decaffeinated coffee or decaffeinated tea with skimmed milk and sugar substitute

Lunch

- South Beach Chopped Salad with Tuna
- Sugar-free jelly

Dinner

- Stir-fry Chicken and Vegetables
- Coleslaw with sesame oil

Dessert

- Lemon Zest Ricotta Crème

DAY THREE

Breakfast

- ½ grapefruit
- Egg white omelette with salsa
- 1 slice multigrain bread
- Decaffeinated coffee or decaffeinated tea with skimmed milk and sugar substitute

Lunch

- Open-faced ham and Swiss cheese sandwich on rye bread
- 1 fresh apple

Dinner

- Grilled sirloin steak
- Creamed Spinach
- Mashed Cauliflower
- Fresh Mozzarella-Tomato Salad

Dessert

- Chocolate-dipped Apricots

DAY FOUR

Breakfast

- ½ grapefruit
- Oatmeal (100g/4 oz old-fashioned oatmeal mixed with 225ml/8 fl oz skimmed milk, cooked on low heat, and sprinkled with cinnamon and 1 tablespoon chopped walnuts)
- 1 poached egg
- 1 slice multigrain bread
- 1 tablespoon low-sugar jam or marmalade
- Decaffeinated coffee or decaffeinated tea with skimmed milk and sugar substitute

Lunch

- Tomato stuffed with chicken salad
- Fresh melon wedge
- 110g (4 oz) fat-free yogurt

Dinner

- Snapper (or Trout) Provençal
- Steamed mange-tout
- Rice pilaf
- Tossed salad (mixed leaves, cucumber, green peppers, cherry tomatoes)
- Olive oil and vinegar to taste or 2 tablespoons low-sugar prepared dressing

Dessert

- Chocolate-stuffed Steamed Pear

DAY FIVE

Breakfast

- ½ grapefruit
- Western Egg White Omelette
- ½ wholemeal muffin
- Decaffeinated coffee or decaffeinated tea with skimmed milk and sugar substitute

Lunch

- Greek Salad
- 110g (4 oz) fat-free raspberry yogurt

Dinner

- Beef, Pepper, and Mushroom Kebabs
- Brown Rice
- Avocado and tomato salad
- Olive oil and vinegar to taste

Dessert

- Almond Ricotta Crème

DAY SIX

Breakfast

- Fresh blueberries
- Cinnamon Surprise
- Decaffeinated coffee or decaffeinated tea with skimmed milk and sugar substitute

Lunch

- Chicken Caesar Salad (no croutons)
- 2 tablespoons prepared Caesar dressing

Dinner

- Savoury Prawns on Wild Rice
- Rocket salad
- 2 tablespoons Balsamic Vinaigrette or low-sugar prepared dressing

Dessert

- Chocolate fondue (made with dark or semi-sweet chocolate) with fresh strawberries

DAY SEVEN

Breakfast

- Fresh orange, sliced
- Tomato and Herb Frittata
- 1 slice multigrain toast
- 1 tablespoon low-sugar jam or marmalade
- Decaffeinated coffee or decaffeinated tea with skimmed milk and sugar substitute

Lunch

- Tuna, Cucumber, and Red Pepper Salad with Lemony Dill Dressing
- Sugar-free jelly

Dinner

- Apricot-glazed Poussins
- Couscous
- Butterhead lettuce salad
- Olive oil and balsamic vinegar to taste or 2 tablespoons prepared low-sugar dressing

Dessert

- Chocolate Sponge Cake

DAY EIGHT

Breakfast

- 150ml (6 fl oz) vegetable juice cocktail
- 1 egg
- 2 slice lean bacon
- ½ wholemeal English muffin
- 1 teaspoonful low-sugar jam or marmalade
- Decaffeinated coffee or decaffeinated tea with skimmed milk and sugar substitute

Lunch

- Grilled chicken salad
- 2 tablespoons Balsamic Vinaigrette or low-sugar prepared dressing

Dinner

- Grilled Rosemary Steak
- Fresh steamed green beans
- Baked Tomatoes with Basil and Parmesan
- Rocket and Watercress Salad
- 2 tablespoons Balsamic Vinaigrette or low-sugar prepared dressing

Dessert

- Fresh strawberries and blueberries in Chocolate Cups

DAY NINE

Breakfast

- Fresh orange, sliced
- 2 Vegetable Quiche Cups To Go
- 1 slice multigrain toast
- Decaffeinated coffee or decaffeinated tea with skimmed milk and sugar substitute

Lunch

- Couscous Salad with Spicy Yogurt Dressing
- Fresh nectarine

Dinner

- Lemony Fish in Foil
- Courgette Ribbons with Dill
- Sliced tomato
- Sliced cantaloupe melon

Dessert

- Strawberries in Balsamic Vinegar

DAY TEN

Breakfast

- ½ grapefruit
- Oatmeal Pancake
- Decaffeinated coffee or decaffeinated tea with skimmed milk and sugar substitute

Lunch

- Open-faced roast beef sandwich (75g/3 oz lean roast beef, lettuce, tomato, onion, mustard, 1 slice granary bread)
- Small Granny Smith apple

Dinner

- Baked chicken breast
- Italian-style Spaghetti Squash
- Tossed salad (mixed leaves, cucumber, green peppers, cherry tomatoes)
- Prepared low-sugar Italian dressing

Dessert

- Sliced nectarines and fresh blueberries with 110g (4 oz) fat-free vanilla yogurt

DAY ELEVEN

Breakfast

- Berry smoothie (225g/8 oz fat-free fruit-flavoured yogurt, 75g/3 oz berries, 75g/3 oz crushed ice; blend until smooth)
- Decaffeinated coffee or decaffeinated tea with skimmed milk and sugar substitute

Lunch

- Frisée and Pecan Salad
- Turkey-tomato pitta (75g/3 oz sliced turkey, 3 tomato slices, handful shredded lettuce, I teaspoonful Dijon mustard in a wholemeal pitta)
- 110g (4 oz) fat-free lemon yogurt

Dinner

- Marinated Grilled Steak
- Grilled asparagus and peppers
- Herb-roasted new potatoes
- Tossed salad (mixed leaves, cucumber, green peppers, cherry tomatoes)
- Olive oil and vinegar to taste or 2 tablespoons low-sugar prepared dressing

Dessert

- Individual Lime Cheesecakes

DAY TWELVE

Breakfast

- ½ fresh grapefruit
- Tex-Mex eggs (2 eggs scrambled with grated Cheddar cheese and salsa)
- 1 slice granary bread, toasted
- Decaffeinated coffee or decaffeinated tea with skimmed milk and sugar substitute

Lunch

- Roast Beef Wrap (Grilled Steak left over from Day 11)
- Fresh nectarine

Dinner

- Grilled salmon with tomato salsa
- Grilled asparagus
- Tossed salad (mixed leaves, cucumber, green peppers, cherry tomatoes)
- Olive oil and vinegar to taste or 2 tablespoons low-sugar prepared dressing

Dessert

- Chocolate-dipped Apricots

DAY THIRTEEN

Breakfast

- ½ grapefruit
- Light Spinach Frittata with Tomato Salsa
- Decaffeinated coffee or decaffeinated tea with skimmed milk and sugar substitute

Lunch

- Red pepper stuffed with cottage cheese and chopped vegetables
- Sliced cantaloupe melon with blueberries

Dinner

- Tandoori Poussins
- Frisée and Pecan Salad
- Couscous
- Hummus with toasted pitta bread and fresh vegetables (you may use ready-made hummus)

Dessert

- Pear poached in dry red wine

DAY FOURTEEN

Breakfast

- South Beach Blintz (1 egg beaten with 75g (3 oz) crumbled cottage cheese and sugar substitute to taste, fried in non-stick omelette pan with cooking spray).
- Decaffeinated coffee or decaffeinated tea with skimmed milk and sugar substitute

Lunch

- Chef's salad (at least 30g (1 oz) each ham, turkey, and low-fat Swiss cheese on mixed leaves)
- Olive oil and vinegar to taste or 2 tablespoons low-sugar prepared dressing
- 1 slice granary bread

Dinner

- Lime-baked Fish
- Grilled Tomatoes
- Steamed Brussels sprouts
- Artichoke salad (chilled cooked artichoke hearts with halved cherry tomatoes and chopped spring onions)
- 2 tablespoons Balsamic Vinaigrette or low-sugar prepared dressing

Dessert

- Chocolate-dipped Strawberries

phase 3 recipes

Once you've reached your goal you'll switch to these recipes, which now include foods such as multigrain bread, tortillas and brown rice. At this point you'll know which carbs you can eat without gaining weight, so you'll have already integrated them into your diet. You'll notice that by this phase we've put an end to the 2 daytime snacks – by now you shouldn't really need them any longer to keep you satisfied between meals. But this is also the phase that includes Chocolate Sponge Cake, which is a fair trade.

BREAKFASTS

TOMATO AND HERB FRITTATA

Serves 2

1 tablespoon Fry Light extra-virgin olive oil cooking spray
110g (4 oz) chopped plum tomatoes
30g (1 oz) chopped spring onions
3 basil leaves, chopped
1 tablespoon low-fat butter substitute
4 eggs, beaten

Coat an ovenproof 30cm (10-inch) frying pan with cooking spray and place over a medium heat until hot. Sauté the tomatoes, spring onions, and basil in the butter until tender. Reduce the heat to low; pour the eggs evenly into the frying pan over the mixture. Cover and cook for 5–7 minutes or until cooked on the bottom and almost set on the top. Transfer the frying pan to a grill and grill until the top is set, 2–3 minutes. Slide onto a serving dish; cut into wedges to serve.

Nutrition at a Glance

Per serving: 169 calories, 16g protein, 5g carbohydrates, 9g fat, 2g saturated fat, 278mg sodium, 1mg cholesterol, 1g fibre

CINNAMON SURPRISE

Serves 1

50g (2 oz) low-fat cottage cheese
1 slice multigrain bread
Peach cinnamon

Spread the cottage cheese onto the slice of bread. Sprinkle with the cinnamon and grill until bubbly, 2–3 minutes.

Nutrition at a Glance

Per serving: 87 calories, 9g protein, 12g carbohydrates, 1g fat, 0g saturated fat, 347mg sodium, 5mg cholesterol, 3g fibre

LUNCHES

COUSCOUS SALAD WITH SPICY YOGURT DRESSING

Serves 4

Couscous

    1 tablespoon extra-virgin olive oil
    1 small onion, finely chopped
    1 small rib celery, finely chopped
    250g (9 oz) couscous
    400ml (14 fl oz) water

Spicy Yogurt Dressing

    3 tablespoons fresh lemon juice
    3 tablespoons fat-free plain yogurt
    1 tablespoon extra-virgin olive oil
    2 teaspoons grated fresh root ginger
    1 clove garlic, crushed
    1 teaspoon ground cumin
    1 teaspoon ground coriander
    Pinch freshly ground black pepper

Salad

    75g (3 oz) dried currants or raisins
    75g (3 oz) tinned chick peas, rinsed and drained
    75g (3 oz) chopped red pepper
    75g (3 oz) chopped green pepper
    2 tablespoons chopped fresh coriander or parsley
    2 tablespoons sliced medium spring onions
    1 lemon, cut into wedges (optional)

To make the couscous: Heat the oil in a 2-litre (4-pint) saucepan over medium heat. Add the onion and celery and cook for 2–3 minutes, stirring occasionally, until the vegetables are softened. Stir in the couscous to coat with oil; cook and stir 1 minute until lightly toasted. Add the water; bring to a boil, stirring gently. Remove from the heat; let stand, covered, for 30 minutes until cool and the liquid is absorbed, uncovering occasionally to fluff with a fork.

To make the spicy yogurt dressing: In a large bowl, mix together the lemon juice, yogurt, oil, root ginger, garlic, cumin, coriander, and pepper. Whisk before serving.

To make the salad: Transfer the couscous to a large serving bowl; spoon the currants or raisins, chickpeas, red pepper, green pepper, coriander or parsley, and spring onions into separate mounds around the couscous. Serve with the dressing. Toss all the ingredients together at the table; garnish with the lemon wedges, if using.

Nutrition at a Glance

Per serving: 393 calories, 12g protein, 69g carbohydrates, 9g fat, 1g saturated fat, 31mg sodium, 1mg cholesterol, 8g fibre

FRISEE AND PECAN SALAD

Serves 6

3 handfuls loosely packed round lettuce
I onion, sliced
3 handfuls loosely packed frisée
¼ teaspoon freshly ground black pepper
90g (3 oz) coarsely chopped pecans, toasted
50ml (2 fl oz) red wine vinegar
¼ teaspoon salt

Combine the lettuce, onion, frisée, and pepper in a large bowl; set aside. Add the pecans, vinegar, and salt to a frying pan and cook over low heat until thoroughly heated. Pour over the lettuce; toss gently.

Nutrition at a Glance

Per serving: 118 calories, 2g protein, 7g carbohydrates, 10g fat, 1g saturated fat, 101mg sodium, 0mg cholesterol, 3g fibre

TUNA, CUCUMBER, AND RED PEPPER SALAD WITH LEMONY DILL DRESSING

Serves 4

Lemony Dill Dressing
    50ml (2 fl oz) extra virgin olive oil
    3 tablespoons fresh lemon juice
    1–2 tablespoons chopped fresh dill
    ½ teaspoon salt
    ½ teaspoon coarsely ground black pepper

Salad
    1 medium cucumber, chopped
    1 red pepper, chopped
    2 tins (185g/6½ oz each) white tuna chunks, drained and flaked
    Romaine lettuce
    1 small lemon, peeled, seeded, and sliced

To make the lemony dill dressing: Whisk the olive oil, lemon juice, dill, salt, and black pepper together in a small bowl.

To make the salad: Combine the cucumber, pepper, and tuna in a large bowl. Set aside. Arrange the lettuce on 4 plates. Spoon the tuna mixture into the centre of each plate. Arrange the lemon around the plates. Drizzle with the dressing.

If preferred, the tuna can be substituted with fresh tomatoes.

Nutrition at a Glance

Per serving: 282 calories, 24g protein, 9g carbohydrates, 17g fat, 3g saturated fat, 640mg sodium, 39mg cholesterol, 2g fibre

ROAST BEEF WRAP

Serves 4

50g (2 oz) low-fat cream cheese
4 × 22–30cm (9–10-inch) flour tortillas
½ red onion, sliced
4 spinach leaves, washed
225g (½ lb) sliced roast beef

For each wrap, spread a small amount of the cream cheese over the surface of a tortilla. Layer the onion, spinach, and roast beef on top; fold in opposite sides of the tortilla about 4cm (1½ inches) and roll up from the bottom.

Nutrition at a Glance

Per serving: 300 calories, 13g protein, 42g carbohydrates, 9g fat, 3g saturated fat, 659mg sodium, 21mg cholesterol, 3g fibre

DINNERS

MOROCCAN GRILLED CHICKEN

Serves 4

50ml (2 fl oz) extra-virgin olive oil
1 teaspoon dried oregano
½ teaspoon ground allspice
½ teaspoon ground cumin
½ teaspoon ground cloves
3 cloves garlic, finely chopped
4 boneless, skinless chicken breast halves
175g (6 oz) couscous
Red Pimiento Sauce

Combine the oil, oregano, allspice, cumin, cloves, and garlic in a large bowl. Add the chicken breasts and cover with the olive oil mixture. Cook on a preheated grill over medium heat for about 30 minutes or until the juices run clear when the chicken is pierced. Remove from the grill and keep warm.

Meanwhile, prepare the couscous according to directions on the packet. When the couscous is ready, divide it among 4 plates; thinly slice each chicken breast and fan over the couscous on each plate. Drizzle 2 tablespoons of the sauce over each chicken breast.

Nutrition at a Glance

Per serving: 429 calories, 32g protein, 37g carbohydrates, 16g fat, 2g saturated fat, 89mg sodium, 66mg cholesterol, 4g fibre